Back On Track

Back ON Track

The Lifestyle & Exercise Guide on Healing Back Pain

Roberta Bergman

Disclaimer

The author is not a medical professional. The theories and exercises are based on the author's research and experience in the field of health, wellness, fitness and movement therapy. The reader is advised always to consult with a medical professional before embarking upon any exercise program.

Published 2024 by Gildan Media LLC
aka G&D Media
www.GandDmedia.com

Front cover design by David Rheinhardt of Pyrographx

Interior design by Meghan Day Healey of Story Horse, LLC

Library of Congress Cataloging-in-Publication Data is available upon request

ISBN: 978-1-7225-0647-6

10 9 8 7 6 5 4 3 2 1

Contents

I dedicate this book to my beloved mother, Jean. She was the most devoted, supportive woman in my life. She inspired me to write this book. Her majestic posture, graceful demeanor, and elegance are her legacy. She taught me how to handle life's most stressful experiences with grace.

I'm grateful to my parents for their pride and love and for always encouraging me to do what I love best.

Foreword

by Aubrey A. Swartz, MD Pharm D

The interest, education, and research in back pain over the past quarter century has been revolutionary. We have discovered a great deal about this very common ailment and about therapeutic possibilities on many levels. We have become increasingly aware that the problems we deal with in back pain are often not just mechanical but are intricately related to the whole person, including their physiology, biochemistry, and psyche. We have come to realize that conditioning and general good health contribute to prevention, in addition to being a part of the treatment.

The health care community has become increasingly aware that important contributions in diagnosis and treatment of back pain have been made by a variety of disciplines, professions and specialists. Increasingly, we realize that we cannot function independently. There is great knowledge to be gained from our unique and varying skills, experience, and training. Over the past few years, clinics and spine centers have developed to provide a more comprehensive level of care to back pain sufferers. We now have interdisciplinary scientific meetings where a diverse group of health care providers come together to exchange information.

Roberta Bergman Haselkorn, founder of the body-formula method, recognizes the direction that back care has taken over the past several years. The information she presents here adopts a practical and understandable clinical approach and makes it enjoyable and meaningful. The current concepts represent the thinking of several leaders in the back care communities. The author has devoted many years of hard work to learning these concepts, which are taught worldwide. Her informative publication should help many people.

This is a self-help book. *Back on Track* will guide the reader through a variety of exercises and movement lessons that will help relieve pain and strengthen and stretch the back. Visual presentations show readers how to find the proper movement method that fits their particular problem. They will learn to distinguish between the various movement forms and decide which one is most suitable. *Back on Track* is not a one-size-fits-all approach. It is a learning tool for people who want to find the right physical technique to heal their back.

I commend Roberta Bergman for her intelligent and practical approach to the prevention and treatment of back pain.

*   *   *

Dr. Swartz, executive director of the internationally acclaimed American Back Society, has twenty-seven years of experience evaluating and treating orthopedic injuries and disease. He led a team of spinal surgeons to Croatia to provide surgical treatment for Bosnian war casualties.

Introduction

———•———

So, Goldie, when did your granddaughter start to exercise so feverishly?" It was a question my ninety-seven-year-old grandmother was asked over and over. She would tell the story: "When Roberta was seven years old, she'd come home from school, put her books down, and exercise. Her sister would always scream at her, 'Get away from me, you're sweating.'"

I was born to move. No wonder. I used to watch my grandmother exercise along with Jack LaLanne's fitness TV show. Granny was a major influence early on.

Like a signature, my pattern of healthy living began during childhood. My priorities were clear.

My body had top priority. Exercise first, then homework, then piano.

I carry my childhood passions with me. I trained as a movement therapist, exercise instructor, personal trainer, and aqua instructor so I could teach other people the joy of feeling fit, strong, and connected to their body.

When I start to work with a new client, I always ask these questions: What are your priorities in terms of your physical body? Where do you place your body in terms of career and family obligations and personal growth?

Often, people forget they have a body. So I keep asking: how do you expect to fulfill your career, family, and personal responsibilities if your breathing is erratic, your body lacks energy, you're mentally fatigued and physically exhausted, you're so stressed that you resent everyone who needs you, and your back is aching to the point where you're unable to work, sleep, enjoy sex, or take part in family activities?

My point usually becomes clear. Until you discharge stress, release your pain, and feel at home in your own skin, you won't be giving your all to anyone, especially yourself. Yes, indeed, you can work with less than full potential, fulfill all your responsibilities with little energy, and walk around with chronic back pain while maintaining a semblance of order. But imagine how much greater your concentration would be if your body was physically fit and in harmony with your mind.

I encourage my students to put themselves on their own VIP list. We examine ways to prioritize health and well-being every day.

Most of us desire physical and mental wholeness, yet we are unwilling or unable or unconscious of the changes necessary to improve our current condition. Why? The answer is simple: the task seems so overwhelming that we become frozen in old patterns.

We go with what we know.

Guess what? There's nothing wrong with taking baby steps. I encourage you to begin today. Small, incremental decisions in exercise habits create the greatest impact over time.

NOTE: If any of the following exercises are painful, please stop immediately!

Chapter 1
Back Pain: Overview and Anatomy

The important thing in science is not so much to obtain new facts as to discover new ways of thinking about them.
—Sir William Bragg

My healthy back philosophy was formed after years of studying the back. Why the back? Most people don't realize that a healthy back is part and parcel to mind and body wellness. Considering that eight out of ten people will experience back and/or neck pain at some point in their lives, it's time we paid attention to our spines.

People from all walks of life are vulnerable to back pain. It spares no one, from couch potatoes to elite athletes. Most notably, back pain is a major complaint with type A personalities. Overachieving, ambitious, worrying, and perfectionism often place stress somewhere, and it is usually in the back.

Most incidents can be related to long-term patterns including poor posture, stressful living, sedentary lifestyles, arthritis, sports injuries, prolonged sitting, poor flexibility, weak muscles, and even repressed emotions. Sound familiar?

Yet back pain continues to be a mystery. Unlike other chronic diseases, it corresponds to no objective or neurological findings in 90 percent of people who suffer. The good news: most back pain can often be alleviated, if not healed, with simple relaxation and medically safe exercise techniques.

This is why I am constantly preaching; "Take your back seriously, and it will take care of you."

Before you wind up in bed over a bad back, let's gain an understanding of how to avoid being a statistic.

Why It Happens

Back pain is proportional to your level of fitness. If your muscles, ligaments, and joints aren't tuned for movement, even something as simple as bending over to tie your shoe can send your back into spasm. Fact is, pain attacks the areas in your body that are the weakest and most vulnerable—the neck and back.

Back pain affects your entire life and can be considered an element of an unhealthy life style. It can cause loss of work, loss of leisure time and sports, low morale, low motivation, low self-esteem, and curtailed sexual activity. Let's face it: when you are in pain and can't engage in your usual routines, you can become overly dependent on others. The result is a loss of independence and stress on your relationships. If your pain isn't that serious, at the very least you lose efficiency.

When you have back pain, any activity, even sex, can be potentially painful and even frightening. How unsettling to be deprived of life's greatest pleasures!

Finally, pain can cause a loss of sleep, which can throw your whole system off balance. Chronic lack of sleep can lead to high stress levels.

Unfortunately, people become immobilized by back pain. It's what I call the "vicious pain cycle." The pain occurs, so you stop exercising and become sedentary.

Pain is an alarm signal; it is not a signal to stop moving. Early activity (within the limits of pain tolerance) is my philosophy. It becomes more difficult and painful to move after extended periods of immobility.

I implore you to take an active role in treating your back pain! It is perpetuated by remaining sedentary: the body becomes disassociated from itself. There is no quick cure for long-term relief of pain. However, specialized exercise is a proactive approach to an active lifestyle.

Exercise is an active ingredient in both healing and preventing back pain. Regular exercise, tailored to your condition, can decrease dependence on health professionals and put the power in your own hands. Stretching, strengthening, aerobics, and relaxation will keep you strong, resilient, and active.

Movement is an active approach to creating a healthy lifestyle. Taking greater care of your body is your best self-defense.

The Big Excuse

I call it *exorphobia*. I have heard everything from "It hurts " to "I don't have the time" to "I think I need to relax" to "I'm too tired." Tired, lazy, stressed-out—regardless of your excuse, I don't buy it.

If we all took our bodies as seriously as our careers, relationships, or families, commitment to exercise would not be an issue. Your body is your business! Exercise improves your personal life, work life, and sex life. My tried-and-true rule: break a sweat three times a week, and stretch every muscle and joint in your body every single day. When we travel by air, we're instructed to put an oxygen mask on ourselves first (before our children or older companions). This is a survival lesson. By taking care of yourself, you can attend to those who need you. YOUR BODY COMES FIRST!

Action, Motivation, Decreased Pain

There are times when even I, the fitness fanatic, don't feel like working out. But I do it anyway, knowing that it's good for my body, attitude, and self-esteem. I try to practice what I preach most of the time and continually aspire to a healthier, fitter, and more active way of life.

I've laid out the facts for you. The problem is not knowledge; it's compliance. Physicians fret when their patients don't follow the rules. Trainers are frustrated when their clients don't follow their exercise regimes. There's always an excuse. You promise yourself that you'll do your back exercises tonight. Tonight comes along and your kids need help with their homework. OK, fine. You'll wake up early tomorrow and do them for sure. Next morning, you sleep through the alarm, and you're off and running. OK, you swear you'll do those exercises after work. The end of the day rolls around. Your boss insists you stay late to finish a project. Your back starts to ache. And on and on . . . The result is obvious. Your back has lost priority.

Make your back number one on your list, and get into action. Say no to every excuse except your back exercises. I'm sure everyone would prefer to have you out of pain.

You don't start out motivated. The action comes first; motivation follows. After your pain decreases as a result of your disciplined practice, motivation will become a reflex. The cycle is action–motivation–decreased pain–motivation–action. It's a positive, reliable chain of events. This cycle will ultimately decrease the number and duration of annual back pain episodes.

The Back Pain Personality

Research has shown that chronic pain patients who have an optimistic outlook cope with discomfort from a problem-solving perspective and are more capable of successful behavior changes.

Optimism is simply a matter of shifting from "*won't* power" (I won't change) to "*will*power" (I want to change). Finding the positive and focusing on it will motivate anyone to action.

Don't let back pain become a way of life. What would your life look like if you didn't have the complaint, "Oh, my aching back"?

Methods of Movement for Back Pain Sufferers

When muscles are in spasm or in just plain pain, movement in any direction causes discomfort. Try not to let the symptoms seduce you to inaction.

The Alexander and Feldenkrais methods (see chapter 5) are both therapeutic and medically safe. They help align the body and bring greater body awareness. These methods send new messages to the brain, which in turn sends new messages to your body.

Exercises that maintain your back in the neutral spine position are also wonderful for back pain sufferers. Walking—the number one sport for people with back pain—maintains the cervical (neck), thoracic (upper back), and lumbar (low back) curves, known as the "neutral spine."

As long as you don't experience back pain while walking, it should be part of your daily routine. A twenty- to thirty-minute (minimum) walk each day keeps the good doctor away.

Overall, it is best to begin gradually and increase the level of difficulty according to your pain threshold. If it hurts, don't do it!

Sciatica: The Big Pain

When something presses on the roots of the sciatic nerve or the sciatic nerve itself, it can knock your socks off! Talk about pain! Sciatic pain can radiate down one leg, or both, all the way to the feet. Sciatica can cause partial paralysis in the hamstrings and prevent movements as simple as walking.

The sciatic nerve is the largest nerve in your body. A continuation of nerve roots from the spine, it supplies the muscles of the leg and foot with sensation. In the lower spine, these nerves diverge to form the right and left sciatic nerves. These nerves traverse the back of the pelvis through the pelvic bone to below the buttock and run down each leg. Sciatic nerves supply the muscles with nerves so that they can contract on demand. They supply nerve function to most of each leg.

Sciatica can cause acute and chronic back pain. Problems occur when a herniated or protruding disc presses on the nerve roots. Sciatic pain causes twinges in the back, buttocks, and down the sides and back of the legs or pain, cramping, and a tingling, numb sensation. It often causes numbness in the feet and sometimes loss of muscle tone. The discomfort can radiate from the buttocks all the way down the thigh to the foot. When the sciatic nerve becomes entrapped inside the pyriformis muscle (deeply embedded in the buttocks), a painful condition known as sciatica often results.

The most important relief stretches for sciatica involve the hamstrings, buttocks, and hips. (See the end of this chapter for sciatica relief stretches.)

Early Mobility Is Key

Ninety percent of all back pain problems spontaneously disappear without any specific treatment. Early mobility is key. Numerous medical studies have demonstrated that early activity decreases the pain and improves mobility. On the other hand, prolonged rest, of even two weeks' duration, can lead to depression and cause muscular atrophy.

The solution? Recondition your body as an artist builds a sculpture. Think of your body as a work in progress, never fully perfected. Working with your body is your opportunity to assume responsibility for wellness. Envision yourself active, healthy, and strong!

To prevent acute and chronic back pain, know your body and back, maintain a good balance between rest and activity, use proper body mechanics, improve your work and home environment, maintain strong abdominal and leg muscles, and keep physically fit—for the rest of your life.

Anatomy Lesson

The spinal column consists of twenty-four vertebrae stacked one on top of the other. Discs, the ball bearings of the spine, separate the vertebrae. Each disc consists of a semifluid center or nucleus held together by ligaments. The discs, similar to rubber washers, act as shock absorbers. They are able to alter their shape, thus allowing movement of one vertebra on top of another. The vertebrae and discs are linked by a series of joints to form the lumbar spine, or lower back.

The spinal column is a supportive system of hundreds of muscles, tendons, and ligaments that run from the brain to the base of the spine. The spinal cord is a bundle of nerves which run vertically through the center of the spinal column.

The back extensor muscles run vertically from the upper back to the base of the pelvis. Between the vertebrae there are openings which allow branches of the spinal cord to exit and supply motor function to the muscles and send sensation to the skin and other areas of feeling. It is through these spinal nerves that we can feel temperature, pressure, and pain.

The seven cervical (neck) vertebrae, which support the weight of the head, enable us to turn our necks. The twelve thoracic (trunk) vertebrae, which support the weight of the torso, permit trunk rotation and are the spinal group to which the rib cage is attached. The five lumbar (low back) vertebrae support the pelvis.

The entire spinal column sits on a platform made of five fused vertebrae called the *sacrum*. The immobile sacrum supports the combined weight of all the other spinal vertebrae. The coccyx, or tailbone, is the lowest part of the spine; it protrudes below the sacrum and has no weight-bearing function.

The roots of the lumbar nerves are the largest of all the spinal nerves. The lumbar area, with the largest vertebrae and the most common site of pain, takes on the greatest stresses and strains in the spine. When your lumbar muscles are strong and flexible, they allow for greater bending movement. When they're taut, the opposite is true.

Movement can stimulate the flow of blood and fluids that nourish the disc, helping to restore its shape. Walking is a wonderful form of exercise to improve circulation and oxygen to the spine. Walking is also great for proper spinal alignment because it maintains the three natural curves in the spine—the neutral spine.

Belly and Buttocks

It's imperative that you build a strong body to protect your back from damage and pain. Your muscles do countless things for you. You use them when you walk, when you lift your child, when you sit in a chair, when you play an instrument or sport, and when you enjoy sex. When you ignore your muscles, they underperform for you and will collapse under pressure. Regular, medically safe exercise, done with proper form, can prevent back problems due to weak muscles. You give your back a boost when your belly and buttocks are strong and in good shape.

We have four sets of abdominal muscles, which form a corset-like appearance. The rectus abdominis runs up and down the abdominal wall. The internal and external obliques run diagonally upward and downward, like pants pockets. Transverse abdominals, or the breathing muscles, run horizontally across the abdomen. These muscles are not isolated: they are layered over one another to work together. We use all our abdominals in tummy exercises.

We need to engage the abdominal muscles, known as the core muscles, to have a positive impact on the lower back. Muscles work in opposition. By strengthening the abdominal muscles in the front, we automatically relax the muscles in the back. So when we strengthen and contract the abdominal muscles, we lengthen, stretch, and relax the back muscles.

When you engage your abs and keep them strong, you position your pelvis properly. In other words, whether you are lifting a bag of groceries, picking up a child, or getting out of a car, engage your core muscles and pull them in to support your back. Use your thighs for support to avoid overrelying on the back muscles.

Core training comes from the inside out and involves facilitating the transverse abdominis and activating the spinal erector. These two muscle groups comprise the core muscles. Drawing in the stomach engages the transverse abdominis. The diaphragm is the chief breathing muscle and is necessary for this process to occur. Breathing awakens your diaphragm, and taking slow, deep breaths allows your belly to expand and contract with each breath. When you exhale, you draw in the core.

If your abs are weak and overstretched, your back extensor muscles are tight and contracted. This underconditioned muscular state can result in a posterior pelvic tilt, known as *lordosis*. This leads to back pain.

Lordosis, or back arching, is a condition that gets more painful overtime. Pregnancy and pot bellies are shoe-ins for back pain. Consider this: every ten pounds of weight places 100 pounds of pressure on the lumbar discs. That's an enormous amount of weight on the lower back.

The weight of the belly arches the back. That's why 65 percent of all pregnant women (or anybody with a paunch) are at risk for back pain. The good news: posture and back exercises can counteract and prevent the painful effects of this postural misalignment.

The quadriceps (the front of the thighs) aid in lifting. If they are not strong, the poor abused back muscles once again take the brunt. The gluteal muscles, the largest muscle group in the body, help support the wiry back muscles. If they aren't strong, we overrely on the back muscles to do the work of the whole body. That's why things pop! To strengthen both the quads and gluteus, you can simply walk.

Caution: Avoid self-diagnosis. See a physician before becoming your own expert.

Chronic Back Pain

Chronic back pain is a long-standing condition that is often debilitating. Chronic back pain can turn sitting, bending, playing sports, working, sex, and walking into *agony*. This kind of nagging pain may bother you periodically.

Statistics show that strained tendons and ligaments cause 80 percent of chronic back pain. It makes sense that regular, medically safe exercise can help mitigate pain.

In fact, physicians do not usually recommend prolonged rest (more than two days) for chronic low back pain.

The "reversibility principle" applies well in this case: "If you don't use it, you lose it." If you are suffering from chronic or acute back pain and don't get proper rest, you can reinjure yourself and set up a recurrent pattern. Going back to life partially recovered with a loss of flexibility, anxiety, and tension is unwise. Early mobility is recommended with therapeutic exercise administered by a physical therapist or a fitness trainer with education in back care. Chronic back pain can last up to seven weeks or more.

Babying your back is not an option. Nursing your back to health is the best way to go. EXERCISE IS THE ANTIDOTE!

Acute Back Pain

Acute pain is of sudden onset, from an injury, a fast, jarring movement, or a twist. It can last up to seven days. Rest is most often prescribed for this kind of pain. However, studies have demonstrated that early activity decreases pain and ensures a quicker recovery.

Treatments for Chronic and Acute

There are two different treatment approaches for chronic and acute back pain.

The treatment for chronic back pain is customized exercise, such as flexion/extension, stretching, strengthening, posture techniques; biofeedback and behavior modification to promote good body mechanics; and relaxation techniques to release tense muscles. The Feldenkrais Method (which I will discuss later) has been known to heal chronic low back pain. It's slow and gentle enough for you to feel pain and stop the movement short of pain. It helps detect changes in your mobility and differentiate the upper, middle, and lower back. This is something we rarely do in the normal course of a day, when the torso is virtually fixed in one position. Feldenkrais movement lessons are geared to use all the joints, muscles, and bones in a way that enhances flexibility for the entire spine. After doing a few movements you will feel as if you have been massaged.

Acute pain is accompanied by tissue damage and is treated very differently than chronic pain. When a nerve root is compressed, it sends pain signals to the brain. You may not be able to walk. One to three days of bed rest, analgesics, and supervised exercise such as soft tissue manipulation by a physical therapist are the medical treatment protocol.

I can't emphasize enough that bed rest is not always the solution. Early mobility is!

Eighty-five percent of chronic lower back pain can be alleviated and prevented if you maintain a balance of strength, flexibility, proper body mechanics, excellent posture, and relaxed muscles. STRONG BODY! TOUGH MIND!

Discs

Discs are the cushions between the vertebrae. They absorb shock. They are enclosed by a tough, fibrous outer shell encasing a thick fluid. The fluid is the shock absorber.

Disc degeneration is part of the natural aging process. Some discs, especially those at the lower end of the spine and the neck, wear out in your twenties. The discs get fatter, suggesting that fluid inside has dried up or broken through a weakened part of the disc wall. As a result, the bones rub together and rub off the padding, creating a ruptured or herniated disc. People think that the discs cause pain. Not true: the soft tissues surrounding the discs produce the pain.

Disc degeneration is regarded as part of the aging process, reflected by the narrowing of disc space or by bony changes. Increasing deterioration of lumbar discs is associated with increasing incidence of back pain. Again, a healthy regimen of exercise can counteract degeneration. So take my ninety-seven-year-old grandmother's advice: "Stop kvetching and start stretching!"

Herniated Discs

Disc herniation, bulging discs, and disc degeneration all cause back and/or neck pain. Pain often defies definition. Research shows that only approximately 20 percent of all acute back pain sufferers can be given a precise diagnosis. We do know that stretching lubricates the joints and brings nourishment to the discs. That's why the Rx for back pain is exercise—strength, mobility (stretching), cardiovascular fitness, and relaxation techniques.

A disc bulges when it loses its ability to absorb shock. The outer wall becomes weakened, and it bulges out. It is similar to squeezing toothpaste from a tube. The fluid does not always break through but may merely bulge through the wall. When the disc bulges far enough out, it may press painfully on the sciatic nerve.

A bulging disc may become severely distorted and prevent the vertebrae from lining up properly during movement. In this case, movement may be painful. It is critical to find a form of movement that will not increase pain. Although yoga and traditional stretching have helped many people, they may actually aggravate a back problem. The Feldenkrais Method is suitable for any chronic condition. The movements are slow and gentle enough to detect pain and isolate the problem.

Inflammatory Back Pain

Inflammatory back pain occurs in 3 percent of the population. It presents itself as spinal inflammation, joint arthritis, and inflammation at the bony insertions. Inflammation can affect the eyes, heart, lungs, skin, mucous membranes, nerves, and kidney.

Various forms of inflammatory back pain are:

Rheumatoid Arthritis

Rheumatoid arthritis is an inflammatory disease that can produce lower back and occasional thigh pain. Night pain is a frequent complaint, but morning pain and stiffness are also reported.

Ankylosing spondylitis, a form of rheumatoid arthritis, is a chronic inflammatory disease accompanied by intermittent low back pain and stiffness. Ankylosing spondylitis is marked by a loss of spinal motion.

Spondylolisthesis

The term *spondylolisthesis* comes from the Greek verb *olisthánein*, meaning *to slip*. Spondylolisthesis is a forward slipping of one vertebra on top of another. It is an abnormality in which two vertebral bones, usually at the end of the spine, are not correctly aligned. This condition is usually present in younger people.

Spinal Stenosis

This generally affects an older age group, typically in their seventies. It is a narrowing of the opening of the vertebrae where the nerves enter. Stenosis is often accompanied by back pain that initially decreases with activity, and eventually recurs. Unfortunately, spinal stenosis is sneaky and recurs often.

Water and Joint Pain

Studies have found a connection between water intake and back and joint pain. According to researcher Dr. Fereydoon Batmanghelidj, chronic pain, such as from arthritis, indicates dehydration.

If the body needs to use water, it draws from the well inside its cells. But when the cells run dry, there is no storage system to draw on. If it takes water from the muscles or joints, this causes what we call dehydration. Dehydration equals *pain*.

Regular water intake is a necessity for those who suffer from arthritis or low back pain. Feel a little achy? Drink water! Even if you're not thirsty, get into the habit of drinking four eight-ounce glasses a day. I challenge you to try it for one week. Measure the results in terms of joint and back pain reduction.

MRI

Magnetic resonance imaging (MRI) is a comparatively new imaging modality for spine disease. Some people prefer it to computerized tomograph (CT) scanning because it lacks radiation exposure. MRI is probably the diagnostic tool of choice for patients with disc problems as well as for diagnosing spinal disorders.

Exercises for chronic pain and sciatica

Day 1.

Legs Up on Chair

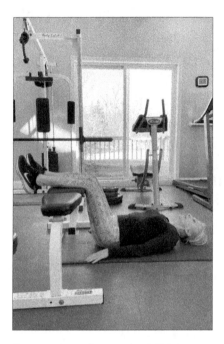 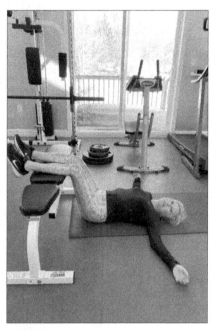

Step 1. Lie on floor, raise both legs up, and rest calves onto a chair or couch. Press lower back down toward floor, arms and shoulders relaxed. Head centered. Relax the back, taking pressure off the spine.

Step 2. Stretch arms outward. Drop your head right and left to relax the neck muscles.

Pelvic Lift

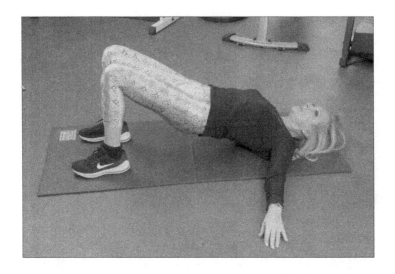

Step 1. Lift hips up to shoulders.

Step 2. Lower to floor by rolling down the spine leading upper back first, then middle back, then lower back last. Repeat sequence a few times.

Day 2.

Sciatic Stretch Sequence

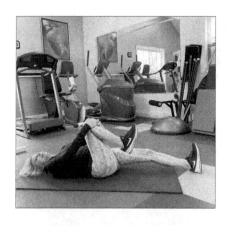

Step 1. Lie on back. Pull one knee over chest, hands below knee, to stretch the hamstring. Hold 10 seconds.

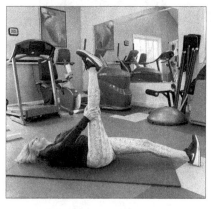

Step 2. Extend same leg straight upward to ceiling; hold hands behind thigh; hold stretch 10 seconds.

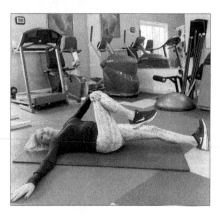

Step 3. Bend the knee, holding the opposite hand on outside of knee.

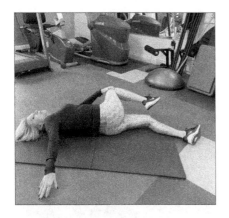

Step 4. Drape the bent knee to opposite side and hold toward floor as far as possible without pain, stretching the sciatic nerve; the other arm is in an outstretched position.

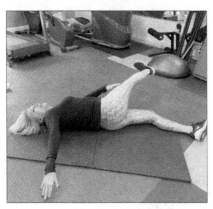

Step 5. Stay on this side; slowly extend the lower leg to straighten the entire leg (toes toward nose). This sequence stretches the sciatic nerve from buttock to ankle. Repeat sequence on other side.

Day 3.

Cat Back Stretch Sequence

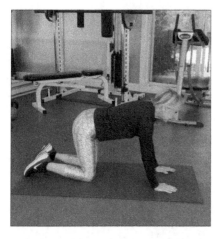

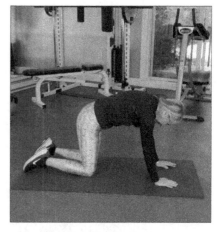

Step 1. Come to hands and knees in flat back position.

Step 2. Round the back, tuck chin to chest, exhale; then arch the back, lift head up, and inhale. Repeat 4 times.

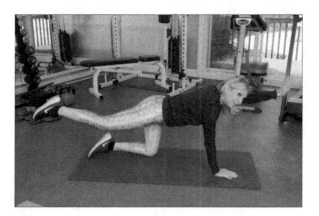

Step 3. On hands and knees, simultaneously extend one arm straight out in front, and extend opposite leg straight out and back. Alternate sides, and repeat the sequence 4 to 8 times on each side. Keep core muscles lifted. This strengthens low back, gluteal muscles, (buttocks), and core.

Back Extension

This four part sequence strengthens back extensor muscles and relieves back pain.

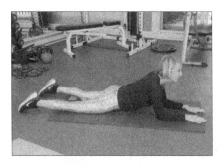

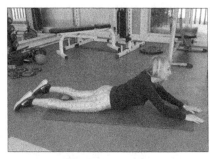

Step 1. **Sphinx.** Lie prone (on stomach), lift chest up to rest on elbows and forearms, hold 10 seconds.

Step 2. **Back pushups.** Lift elbows off floor, straighten arms, hold 4 seconds, then lower elbows to floor. Exhale while straightening arms. Repeat 10 times. (Stop if painful.)

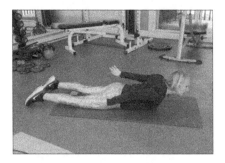

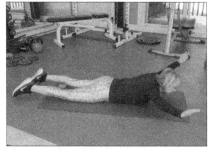

Step 3. **Airplane stretch.** Bring arms behind body, lifted off floor. Raise legs and arms off floor, airplane position. Hold 4 seconds, then lower body to floor. Repeat several times.

Step 4. **Superman stretch.** Bring arms straight out front and lift arms and legs simultaneously off the floor. Hold position 4 seconds, then lower to floor. Repeat 8 times.

Chapter 2
The Five Common Causes of Back Pain

Learning is not attained by chance; it must be sought
for with ardor and attended to with diligence.
—ABIGAIL ADAMS 1780

There's always something (or someone) to blame back pain on. I've outlined the most common reasons for your pain. Identify yourself in any of the following five areas, and you're ahead of the game: improper posture, under-conditioned muscles, stress, incorrect body mechanics, and prolonged sitting.

Bad Posture = Bad Back

Who would think that the most common cause of back pain is poor posture? But consider this: your head weighs between ten and fourteen pounds. If it migrates even an eighth of an inch forward, it becomes a thirty-pound weight. So how often do we walk around looking at the ground and slumping forward? The weight of your head is enough to throw your whole spine out of alignment! It's no wonder your neck feels tense and painful at the end of a day.

Even the normal aging process affects posture. As we age, gravity takes the body closer to the ground. The more we give in to gravity, the more slouched we become.

Posture is also affected by long hours of sitting and forward bending. For instance, a mom who hunches while strolling with a carriage all day, a dentist standing over patients, and a car mechanic hanging over a car are prime candidates for neck and back pain.

The result of these dysfunctional poses (shoulders drooped, head jutting forward, chest caved in) is, at the worst, painful kyphosis (rounded shoulders) and at the best, tightness and loss of full range of motion, with rigidity.

Normal lordosis is the natural curvature of the spine, shaped like the letter S. The neck area (cervical spine), curves inward, the upper back (thoracic spine) curves outward and the lower back (lumbar area) curves inward. The three curves form an S-shape. For best posture and back pain prevention, the emphasis is on maintaining these three natural curves.

There are three postural misalignments; lordosis (lower back arching), kyphosis (rounded shoulders with drooping spine) and scoliosis (congenital condition), causing a lateral shifting of the spine.

A condition known as "Postural Lordosis" comes from being overweight, pregnancy and/or lack of muscle conditioning in the lower back and core. The muscles of the core (abdominal muscles) can be weak and the back muscles can be tight and/or weak. This creates a painful condition known as "postural lordosis." When the pelvis tilts forward and the lower back and hips lift up, it creates an exaggerated arching of the lower back along with a protrusion of the abdomen. The back muscles then become too tight. The added weight of the abdomen places increased pressure on the lower back which exacerbates back pain. Postural lordosis also occurs in thin people.

To correct "postural lordosis," tuck the pelvis under to reduce back arching. Also, lift the abdominal muscles in and up to support the spine. It is imperative to strengthen the core and back muscles and stretch tight back muscles. It would also help to lose weight to unload the forces on the spine, knees and hips. To reverse "postural lordosis," perform the exercises on page 34, page 118, and page 143 regularly.

Spine Talk

To recapitulate: a healthy spine is arranged in three curves forming an S shape. The curves are based at the neck (cervical), the middle back (thoracic), and the lower back (lumbar). When properly aligned, these natural curves keep your body balanced and supported in movement. They also distribute your weight evenly throughout your spine, making back injuries less likely.

The lumbar curve is the workhorse of your spine. It is the hardest-working curve in the spine, carries the most weight, and moves the most. Aligning your lumbar curve helps prevent injury to vertebrae, discs, and other parts of your spine.

Learning proper posture is key to proper alignment. Keep the back of your head lifting forward and up, shoulders widened out to the sides and over the hips, with your pelvis and hips hanging loosely underneath you. Picture your head balancing like a balloon with the string hanging down the length of your spine.

To develop good posture, use your full height whether you are sitting, standing, working or walking. Did you ever notice how heads turn when someone with great posture walks into a room? Use your posture to take on a winner stance and look ten years younger! Like any new habit, posture takes practice. Awareness is key. When your muscles, joints, ligaments, and nervous system operate in an integrated manner, movement is agile and spontaneous, and posture is correct.

Pay attention to posture while at your computer, playing tennis or golf, weight lifting, or walking. Correct posture will help you hold a baby, lift an object, and sleep more comfortably.

Remember that you pay the price for poor posture, and you reap the rewards of the proper posture. Keep your posture on your mind!

Strong, Flexible Muscles

Strong, flexible muscles help maintain your three natural curves by holding your vertebrae and discs in proper alignment. When your abdominal, hip, thigh, buttock, and back muscles are toned, they take the strain off your back.

Think of your trunk as a girdle of strength, your base of power. If you're one of those guys who carry extra weight in the "love handles" or a woman who stores it in the midriff, you're putting your back to the task.

Let's talk about this more. The buttocks (gluteal muscles) are the strongest muscles in the body. If you keep them strong with exercises such as squats, lunges, and leg lifts, you are one step further along to a strong back. The belly muscles can also be toned in a variety of ways. Now you are two steps along. These are the two building blocks of your foundation!

For ease of movement, you need to practice simple stretches for the hamstrings, lower back, hips, and shoulders. Tense muscles don't perform as well as strong and flexible ones. My fitness philosophy for a pain-free back is to be as flexible as you are strong. Stretching every day will ensure agility in all movement.

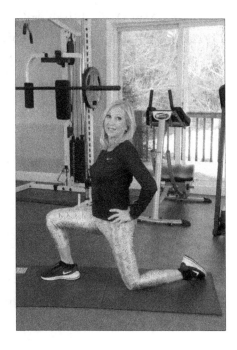

Hip flexor stretch for the iliopsoas muscle (sitting muscle). Place hands on hips and press the pelvis forward to stretch the back thigh. Repeat on both sides (see full sequence on page 142).

Stress and Its Impact on Back Pain

Wouldn't it be great if you could relieve tension by pushing a button on your computer? Your shoulders would instantly drop, your brow would become smooth, your headache would go away, you'd breathe deeply, and your neck pain would vanish.

Stress is insidious and sneaks up on you when you least expect it. It takes many forms, usually beginning with shallow chest breathing as opposed to deep belly breathing. But the detrimental effects of stress are compounded like layers of lasagna. First your jaw clenches (TMJ); then your facial muscles tighten; your shoulders shrug; the pain between your shoulder blades begins; your head aches, next your neck, and then your back. This is very common.

Let's say that to combat all this tension, you go to work out. Now you twist a little too hard or bend a bit too far and, ouch! your back goes out. Blaming the problem on your workout is not the answer. You can blame the problem on stress.

Some of the more common symptoms of stress include erratic and shallow breathing, poor posture, tension headaches, back and neck pain, insomnia and restlessness, cracking knuckles, teeth grinding, excessive fatigue, short temper, muscle tension, and cold hands. When you are physically and mentally exhausted, you are vulnerable. In fact, mental fatigue (often disguised as physical exhaustion) is high on the stress list.

Stress and breathing are inextricably intertwined. Breathing awakens your diaphragm, the breathing muscle. We activate upper chest breathing when under stress, which can lead to chronic stress.

How does all this stress show up? Check it out on your-self. If your back and neck are tight or weak, that is where your pain will go. The good news: you can develop skills to combat stress through the breath. (See chapter 6.)

Prolonged Sitting

Sitting puts a greater strain on the lower back than lying, standing, or walking. Consider this: The seated position places approximately 400 pounds of pressure on your lower back. Standing upright places 175 pounds of pressure on your lower back. Lying flat on your back with your legs extended straight in front of you places only seventy-five pounds of pressure on your low back. Lying on your back with your knees resting on a chair places only twenty-five pounds of pressure on your lower back. THIS IS THE MOST RELAX-ING POSITION FOR YOUR LOWER BACK. This is the best exercise to do when your back is aching. (See chapter 1.)

Most of our work requires long hours of sitting. My advice: Take minibreaks throughout the day. Stand up and stretch whenever you feel your back tighten, when your neck starts to nag at you, or when you notice your posture droop-ing. Get up and walk around frequently to unload your discs and nourish your spine.

Make sure your seated position is correct. Place your back and buttocks against the back of the chair and roll your shoulders backwards. NO SLOUCHING ALLOWED. Another primary effect of spending long periods of time sit-ting is that the hip flexors shorten. If you're at the keyboard or phone, take frequent breaks to stretch the fingers, wrists, forearms, hips, and back. When you feel your mind clouding up, take a few deep, cleansing breaths.

The correct sitting posture is to sit in a straight-back chair, with good lumbar and/or upper back support, using a pillow, a rolled towel, or an ergonomically correct chair. The head should be lifted, shoulders straight, stomach in, and feet flat on the floor. If your sciatica acts up, place your foot (of the leg in pain) on a low stool. If you have adequate support in your lumbar spine, you won't have so much pressure in your neck. Instead of using your shoulders to hold your body, use your entire back. Once again, I recommend the Feldenkrais and Alexander techniques for better body awareness.

The problem with the computer is that the computer screen monopolizes your eyes, so you don't pay attention to your body. Your body goes kaput! Even if you are using minute movements of the fingers, hands, and wrists, you need the support from your center, the torso, and pelvis. Sit at the front edge of your seat, push your chest out, then sink it back. Push the shoulders out, then back a few times.

The key is to change the condition of your torso from postural fixity to postural flexibility. Once the torso becomes rigid and fixed for hours without moving, all sorts of postural misalignments and tensions manifest in the neck, upper back, and low back. Haven't you noticed that at the start of the day you sit tall but by the end of the day, you end up in the classic slouch—belly hanging, shoulders rounded, chest sunken, and head drooped? With some postural awareness, you can remind yourself to move from the center of your body rather than just the extremities.

To prevent the detrimental effects of sitting, take a few moments to slowly stretch the neck, back, arms, and legs before you go to sleep. One way to relieve pressure from the spine is to lie on your stomach on the floor, with a mat underneath. Lift one leg off the floor at a time, holding the leg up for a count of four, and repeat eight times for each side. This exercise can be done anywhere—in a hotel room, at the gym, in your office, or in front of the TV. Something as simple as a back relief exercise can save you from a lifetime of pain!

Ergonomics: An Office Workstation Guide

Ergonomics is the study of your work, home, and/or office environment and how you adapt to it. It takes into consideration your comfort level at your workstation, play station, and kitchen. It involves how you sit in a chair, stand, and maneuver around your job tasks and home activities. Your work environment usually includes your chair, desk light, computer terminal with keyboard and mouse, telephone, calculator, writing tools, paper, books, magazines, catalogs, family pictures, and personal belongings. An unorganized work zone increases stress, pain, and fatigue, obviously affecting your productivity and success. When ignored, little aches and pains turn into chronic discomfort, which can eventually lead to missed work time.

Set up your workstation in a way that makes you feel comfortable. Try different configurations until you find one that fits your body. Ergonomic workstation modifications, posture awareness, and chair consciousness will enable you to be more comfortable throughout the day. Here are some guidelines.

Chair Consciousness

The chair is the most important object at your desk. If you feel shorter at the end of the day, here's why: we lose an inch and a half simply by sitting. The discs between the vertebrae lose water and compress. Sitting without strain is really a challenge. Having an ergonomically correct seat can help alleviate back pain. The most important area of concern is the lumbar area, or lower back. Some chairs have no low back support at all, while others are too flat.

Most people sit at the edge of chairs that are too high for them. This pitches your body forward, throwing it out of alignment.

Approach Your Chair with Ergonomic Modifications

1. Allow your feet to rest firmly on the floor, slightly in front of you. Lean back in the chair, with your lower back close to the back of the chair.
2. Cushioned seats are the best.
3. The back rest should be adjustable for pelvic and lumbar support. Lean back in the chair to redistribute back pressure. Tilting back (reclined) reduces stress on your back. Place a rolled-up towel or lumbar pillow behind your lower back and/or upper back to keep the chest lifted. This prevents sinking into your lower back and maintains an upright posture.
4. Maintain proper adjustments for your chair. If your knees touch your keyboard, your chair is too high. If your feet

cannot rest flat on the floor, use a footrest for one foot or both.

5. Evaluate whether your chair is comfortable for one to two hours. Do this for one week. If it's not comfortable, look for an ergonomically correct chair.

6. Static seated postures are the precursors for back and neck pain. Take frequent stretch breaks to change positions throughout the day.

Maintaining good posture while you sit will help prevent muscular fatigue, drooping shoulders, and pain. When you feel yourself slipping into a pain-inducing posture, simply lift your breastbone and roll your shoulders backward. Use your full height even in a chair.

According to *The Journal of Applied Ergonomics* in 2019, "there is an association between static sitting, sedentary behavior and chronic low back pain." Any static position can be uncomfortable for long periods of time. Every hour, take minibreaks for movement; stand up and arch the back (or sit down if you are standing for long periods), stretch your arms overhead, and then out to the sides for the back and chest. Stretch the wrist flexors and extensors; use shoulder shrugs and circles to release tension in the shoulders. A short walk to another room works wonders for the spine every hour. According to Nancy L. Black, an associate professor who specializes in ergonomics in the department of mechanical engineering at University de Moncton in Canada, "as you sit or even stand, gravity compresses the discs in your back and may cause back pain and nerve issues. Just twenty to thirty seconds of moving around, draws fluid back into the discs. This sets everything back in proper position."

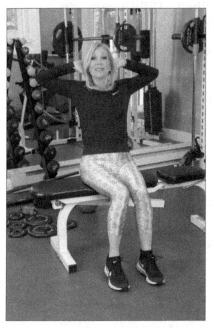

Seated stretch for upper body.

Step 1. Place hands behind the head and pull elbows back to stretch the pectoral muscles of the chest and the rotator cuffs inside the shoulders. Then arch and extend the upper back as if reclining in a chair. This improves and reverses the seated posture.

Step 2. Sit tall, lifting breastbone. Twist to one side, place both hands on the outside seat of a chair, and hold the stretch a few seconds. Stretch the rib cage, waistline, and back.

Step 3. Repeat on the other side.

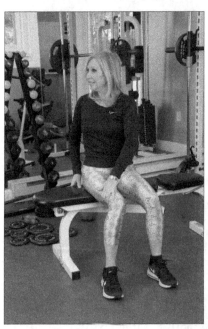

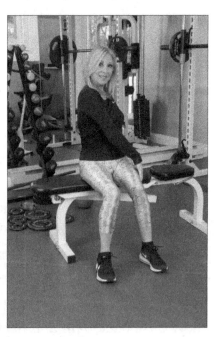

The Keyboard and the Mouse

Most people either twist or strain to reach the keyboard or sit in odd contortions, which eventually leads to neck, back, or wrist pain. Here are some tips for proper positioning of the keyboard and the mouse:

1. Center your keyboard in front of your monitor. Your eyes should be between eighteen and twenty-four inches viewing distance from the screen.
2. Keep the keyboard and mouse as close as possible to the edge of the desk so you don't have to reach for them.
3. Position the keyboard and mouse so that your arms fall naturally at your side, with wrists straight out in front of you, while typing or using the mouse.
4. Support your wrists and forearms with a gel pad or wrist support.
5. Avoid repetitive gripping of the mouse.
6. Place frequently used items within arm's reach. Don't reach for anything!
7. Take frequent stretch breaks!

Keyboard Athletics

This may seem like an oxymoron, but it's a very real dilemma. Just because you're not breaking a sweat while sitting at the computer doesn't mean you're not giving your back a workout. Even if you start your day sitting tall in your chair, by the end of the day you're probably hanging over your keyboard with rounded shoulders and jutted neck. The computer monopolizes your eyes, and your body goes kaput!

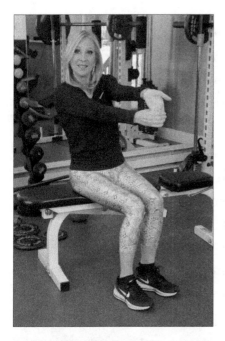

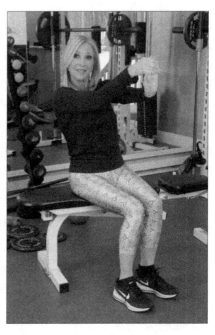

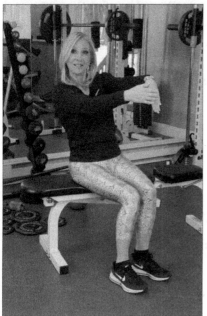

Wrist, Hand, and Finger Stretches

Step 1. Sit tall (breastbone lifted) and extend arm straight out in front, with fingers of one hand pointed down and turned outward. Hold fingers down with the other hand.

Step 2. Reach arm out in front of body (stop sign position). Pull fingers toward face (with other hand) to hold stretch a few seconds, then release.

Step 3. Stretch arm out with top of the hand forward, and press fingers downward with pressure of other hand and fingers. All 3 exercises stretch the forearm and wrist flexors and extensors. It's the perfect stretch break while working.

I cannot emphasize enough how important it is to get into shape. Sitting for hours mesmerized by the screen or standing for extended periods of time requires a team of strong and flexible muscles wrapped around your trunk. Keyboard athletics require as much conditioning as any other sport. Weight lifting will strengthen your postural muscles to help hold your body upright. Abdominal (core) and back exercise will strengthen and protect the back. Lengthening and stretching is an efficient strategy for creating spinal stability and proper posture.

Proper Body Mechanics When Lifting Objects

Low back pain often starts when a heavy object is lifted incorrectly or too suddenly. Think of a forklift picking up a cement block. The angle the forklift uses is 90 degrees, the strongest lifting angle. The same is true for your body. Here are the basics:

When you lift an object, stand with your feet planted at hip width apart, keeping your mind on your posture.

1. As you lift, bend your knees and go down to the object keeping your back straight and upright. Not round!

2. Hold the object close to your body with forearm and upper arm perpendicular. As you lift, straighten knees, and lean back slightly to maintain balance. Lift smoothly.

3. When standing, shift your weight by pivoting the entire pelvis to turn. Don't just twist your back.

4. Take breaks. Make sure you stretch your chest upward to release the pressure of lifting.

As you can see, back pain is not just a matter of flabby abs or a drooping derriere. The problem is multifaceted and requires positive change. You are on your way to self-awareness. Educating yourself about your back is a powerful choice.

Emergency Tip Sheet

In emergency episodes of acute pain, follow these instructions. If any of the steps cause you pain, stop immediately.

Stop. Lie on the floor with your hips close to the legs of a chair and place calves on the seat of the chair.

Rest. Don't exercise for one day. The next day, lie flat on your back and do a few small pelvic tilts every two hours. Roll onto your belly and do a few slow back push-ups every few hours, but only if this position does not cause pain. If it does, discontinue this movement and do only pelvic tilts.

Relax. Breathe mindfully. Take a few deep breaths and exhale slowly. Repeat the following words silently: *relax . . . be still . . . be calm.*

Aspirin, ice, and heating pads. First, consult with your doctor. Then use aspirin, ibuprofen, or Aleve to take down the swelling and relieve the pain. Anti-inflammatory medication can be extremely useful during the acute phase. Next, apply ice packs for twenty minutes every hour until the pain subsides. Follow with alternating cold and heat (nonelectric heating pads are best).

Alternative methods. Homeopathy, acupuncture, herbs, and massage all provide excellent healing properties. Back yourself up with resources.

After the pain. Start a program of exercise to build up your back and abdominal (core) muscles and increase flexibility. Don't get in trouble again!

Chapter 3
Poor Posture and Back Pain

*The spine is your tree of life. Stand up
and keep your back straight.*

—Martha Graham

Posture is like a signature. You established and rein-
forced it during childhood. Were you told to sit up or
stand up straight? Are your shoulders rounded, your back
swayed, your stomach thrust out? Are you jutting your neck
out like a duck or in like a turtle? Were you sick of hearing,
"Pull your shoulders back," "Don't slouch," and so on?

How do you know whether your role models (parents and
teachers) knew the correct posture?

The good news is that you can correct poor posture at
any age. Changing posture habits often feels strange and
awkward. But don't be alarmed. Like all new habits, learning good posture takes time and practice. Remember that it
takes twenty-one days to learn a new habit. Proper posture

will help you look and feel better and reduce back and neck pain and even eye strain.

Fantastic posture will take ten years off your age. Good posture looks majestic and exudes an attitude of confidence and positive body image.

Posture is responsible for the majority of body habits we have developed over the years. Although your signature posture may resemble that of a drooping plant, you may not be aware of your postural habits. They not only look bad, they *are* bad. They cause back pain, neck pain, rounded shoulders, tension headaches, tightness in the jaw, TMJ disorder, eyestrain, and a variety of muscular imbalances and postural misalignments. Poor posture can be a serious and life-damaging condition when ignored and neglected. Fantastic posture is a learned skill integral to changing incorrect posture habits.

Dealing with the inevitability of gravity is a matter of fighting the aging process. As we age, gravity draws our shoulders, head, and neck closer to the floor. Before you know it, your head is hanging on your chest, and the rest of the body slowly cascades down with the rest of the spine like a domino effect. If you don't work your posture, gravity will.

This is 99 percent preventable with posture reeducation. The fault does not lie with gravity or the burden our backs must bear, but with lack of awareness and control of supporting musculature. The relationship between the head, neck, and spine, along with good flexibility in the neck, shoulders, back, hamstrings (back of thighs), calves, and ankles, is critical to good posture. Strength in the abdomen, back, hip flexors, gluteal muscles (buttocks), and the hamstrings, as well as strong upper, middle, and low back muscles, are important to trunk strengthening in order to support the weight of the entire torso.

To change incorrect posture and create fantastic posture, you need discipline and good old-fashioned hard work. How do you get to Carnegie Hall? Practice, practice, practice. Most people get lazy and lose their initial level of exuberant motivation toward changing the condition of their bodies. But it only takes five minutes, three times per day, to reinforce proper posture.

The mirror will give you instant feedback. Remember, instead of your head going out like a duck or in like a turtle, make sure it's centered over your shoulders. Notice the contours of your spine.

Look in a mirror and align your head so that it balances evenly between your shoulders; make sure your shoulders are rolled back, your abdominal muscles lifted, and pelvis in neutral: not too far under, not too arched.

While you're at work, sit at the edge of your seat and simply lift your breastbone. You don't have to force or push your shoulders forward or pull them back. Think about lifting the breastbone upward by placing your index finger on it and lift to your full height. Most people tilt their head too far back or jut the neck too far forward, which throws the entire spine out of alignment. Right now, simply lift the back of the head (not the face!) forward and up so it's held high. Bring the chin slightly into the chest. This will reinforce proper placement of the head and neck.

This action takes the torso off your diaphragm, which enables you to breathe deeply and sit tall. If you're slouched with a caved-in chest, it cuts off the breath. Whenever the flow of breath is obstructed, physical tension (often disguised as mental fatigue) sets in. Learn to use your full height when you sit, stand, and walk. *Keep your posture on your mind all day long!*

Postural Misalignments

The back and trunk muscles accommodate the three natural curves of the spine. As we have seen, these are: (a) the cervical curve of the neck; (b) the thoracic curve of the middle back; (c) the lumbar curve of the lower back. When you maintain these three natural curves in their normal alignment, your weight is evenly distributed through the vertebrae and discs, and your back is less vulnerable to injury.

The proper posture is maintained when your chest is out, chin is tucked, and your ears, shoulders, and hips are in a straight line. Having the pelvis is tilted too far forward causes lordosis of the spine, known as a swayback or arching. This is the first postural misalignment. (By the same token, if your back is tilted too far forward creating an accentuated "flat back," you remove the natural S curve in the spine. This can also lead to back pain.)

When your shoulders droop forward, causing rounded shoulders, the thoracic region of the upper back has an accentuated curve, which is extremely disabling. Most of your energy is spent trying to hold this unsuitable posture rather than utilizing the effort required for an activity. In its extreme form, this is called *kyphosis*, and it is most common in older people. However, the condition begins early on and can be caused by sitting long hours in one fixed position or simply from lack of awareness of proper posture. Kyphosis is the second misalignment.

The last misalignment is scoliosis—a lateral curvature of the spine. Unless it is congenital, scoliosis is caused by a muscular imbalance between the right and left sides of the body. Scoliosis can be corrected 85 percent of the time with muscular conditioning and fantastic posture lessons and Feldenkrais movement lessons (described later).

The Alexander Technique for Correct Posture

About one hundred years ago, a little-known Tasmanian actor named F.M. Alexander lost his voice. His subsequent self-help odyssey evolved into a technique now used worldwide to enhance sports and artistic performance, counter back pain, and complete everyday activities by balancing the body in everyday movement.

Alexander repeatedly found that rest and medical remedies could soothe and restore his voice but couldn't keep him from losing it again. Doctors agreed that the problem must have originated in something he was doing, but they couldn't say what. Through lengthy self-observation, Alexander discovered that when he sang, he distorted his posture, tensing arms and legs, lifting his chest, pulling his head back, stiffening neck muscles, and depressing his larynx enough to impair use of his vocal cords. Eventually Alexander developed a technique to help him and others reeducate their movements to cause the least wear and tear on the body.

The concept of good use of the body, according to Alexander, is to allow your neck to release so that the top of your head can balance forward and up. Allow your back to lengthen and shoulders to widen and expand across your upper back. Allow your shoulders to release out to the sides. Loosen your pelvis by dropping your buttocks down toward your heels without tipping your tailbone too far forward and under or too far backward and arched.

In order to produce clear sound, the head must be in proper alignment with the rest of the spine. If the chest collapses, breathing is impeded and the voice is strained. If the head is off balance, the muscles and spine must contort to keep the body erect. The Alexander technique helps restore the head and spine to their proper balance.

The Alexander Technique does not involve a series of exercises, relaxation training, or psychotherapy. Part of studying the technique is learning how to observe yourself and develop a better, more accurate, and reliable body image.

If your neck is plagued by perpetual tension, occasional pain, and crippling spasms, this method will help you shed long-established habits and learn how to use your body with ease and grace. You learn to work out a new stance and retrain the action of your muscles until you regain control of your posture and even your voice. Whether you read, write, drive, work at a computer, play a musical instrument, cook, sew, garden, play tennis, swim, cycle, dance, sit, stand, walk, talk on the phone, or carry groceries, you unconsciously tense the muscles between your head and upper back. Because most of us no longer harvest hay, churn butter, or gather fruit, we have become more dissociated from the physical body than at any other time in history.

The Alexander method teaches a more relaxed and natural posture. It teaches you how to soften the neck and float the head. Awareness is key.

For more about the Alexander Technique, see chapter 5.

What Is Tech Neck?

Screen technology is the prime culprit of neck pain for preteens, teens, and adults. It has taken over our lives, making the neck the most overused part of the body. Overuse of PlayStations, iPads, computers, and phones all play a role in tech neck.

The head weighs between ten and fourteen pounds. If it migrates forward an eighth of an inch, it becomes a thirty-pound weight, like a bowling ball hanging over your chest. It's enough to throw your entire spine out of alignment, ruin your posture, and instigate neck pain.

As we age, gravity takes the body closer to the ground. Your posture suffers when the head and neck repetitively droop forward over the chest. This postural misalignment, known as kyphosis, is common to people as they age. The head and neck are thrust forward, the shoulders round and stoop forward and the upper back can form a rounded hump (known as a dowager's hump) over time. This condition ranges from young children to older adults.

As the aftereffects of the pandemic persist, many people continue to work remotely from home or a hybrid of office

and home. Since early 2020, the pandemic has forced people to relocate their office to their home. Living rooms, din-
ing rooms, and kitchens have become office spaces. Chairs
and couches are not always ergonomically designed, leaving
many people with stressful body postures that contribute to
back and neck pain. Fingers and hands may tingle from overuse, known as repetitive strain injury. This condition may
lead to carpal tunnel syndrome. Talking on the phone while
keying in information as the phone is cradled awkwardly by
the upper back and neck muscles may also lead to chronic
back and neck pain.

Tips to Avoid and Minimize Tech Neck

1. **Posture.** Keep the lift in the breast bone and back of the
   head while sitting and standing. Place two fingers on the
   breast bone to lift the chest up and off the diaphragm.
   Press one finger on the chin to tuck it in, rather than jutted out. Then press the chin inward so the back of the
   head lifts forward and upward. Be aware of the placement
   of the head. Practice by pulling the back of your head to
   the back of the headrest in your car for correct placement
   of the head.

2. **Line of sight.** Avoid looking down at your screen. Raise
   the device to eye level by placing it higher up. Stack a few
   books or the equivalent and rest the screen there in order
   to keep it at eye level.

3. **Self-awareness.** Keep your posture on your mind at all
   times. Like all new habits, good posture takes awareness,
   practice, and repetition. Use your full height even when
   sitting.

4. **Neck mobility.** Exercise for the neck includes neck stretches and toning, done on a mat on the floor. Lie flat on the floor with your head resting on the floor. Drop your head from right to left and notice which side of the neck is tighter, with less range of motion. Then drop your chin downward toward the chest and release it. Repeat four times. This elongates the neck and reduces pain. Then trace a small plate, leading with your chin, circling four times in one direction, then four times in the other direction. Practice these exercises daily, especially when you notice neck pain.

5. **Pillows.** Try several different pillows until you find one that shapes itself comfortably to both sides of your neck. If the pillow is too stiff, it will place your neck in an awkward position and may result in neck pain when you awaken. Pillows that are too mushy will not provide enough support. Once you find the pillow that's best for your neck, you may notice a remarkable decrease in pain.

Walking Posture

I had the good fortune to participate in David Balboa's Walking System lessons in Central Park in New York City. Students were given a bungee cord tied around their waist that was attached to the trunk of a tree. We were asked to walk away from the tree trunk, let go of the torso, let the arms swing freely, and release the back. It felt very different from regular walking, which often feels held and controlled.

After walking forward and away from the tree, we were then instructed to walk backwards. Since we have no regular experience of walking backwards, we have not formed unchangeable posture habits in this regard. This experience gives you the opportunity to learn a new way of walking. Try walking backwards in a safe open space sometime. Notice the change in your gait and your awareness of your posture.

Many people experience back pain because they are walking with dysfunctional posture. Learning to walk well is one form of back pain prevention. When the posture is slumped, the lower back remains tight and contracted, the hips rigid. The body is pitched forward, breathing is restricted, and movement is confined. Walking in this position can be painful. The most beneficial way to walk is with the posture erect, the lower back relaxed, the hips swinging freely, and easy breathing.

When you walk well you feel as if your whole body has been exercised from your shoulders to your toes. And guess what? No pain afterwards.

Imagine your legs starting at the top of your waistline. When you walk, use your upper body in a counterrotation to your hips. Feel your shoulders move in opposition to your hips, as a model walks down a runway. Exaggerate the movement. It may feel a little affected, but here's your chance to perform and strut your stuff. Of course, you'll tone down the motion in real life. By exaggerating the movement, you'll balance the rigidity in your torso and ignite some motion in the upper body and hips.

Glide as you walk, slow it down, feel the rhythm, and don't bounce. Walking can be a flowing, tension-releasing movement.

Instructions from David Balboa: As your heel contacts the ground, feel that connection firmly. Then roll your foot forward toward your toes and allow your foot to press into the ground. Try the entire heel-to-toe motion. Imagine and feel that the effort of standing tall is coming from the ground up—from your feet and legs, through your abdomen and chest, and finally to your head.

Walking with good posture does more than make someone look self-assured. It reduces stress on the entire body. You'll be able to walk longer, more rhythmically, with grace, and not feel as fatigued. Besides, you never know who'll be admiring your new posture.

Sleep Postures

Yes, it's possible that how you sleep affects how your back feels. The worst way to sleep is flat on your belly. It can take the natural S curve out of your spine. One way to keep the curve is to place a pillow under your tummy to reduce stiffness in your neck. This will help maintain the S curve. But this is still not the optimum position for pain-free sleeping.

Lying flat on your back is better than lying on your belly, although it is not the ideal position for proper sleep alignment either. If your habit is to sleep on your back, use a pillow under your knees to maintain the natural curve and reduce low back pain. If the pillow is not comfortable, adjust its height or shape until you feel a relaxed back. Pillows vary: it's not a "one size fits all." Try a cylinder, oblong, or lumbar pillow until you find the right one to place underneath your knees.

The best sleep position is lying on your side. Your back is in better placement to maintain alignment. If you sleep on your side and still wake up with back pain, place a pillow between your knees and underneath your elbows.

While you sleep, what is called *nuclear fluid* runs through the entire length of your spine. It oozes out and presses against the walls of the discs during the night. That's why you wake up feeling a little stiff in the morning. This also may be why sudden movements in the morning can injure your discs. If you feel stiff, take it slow in the mornings and wait at least an hour until you exercise vigorously. In the evening your body as a rule becomes more flexible. Perhaps this would be the best time for you to exercise, especially if you have back problems.

During the day, fluid is pushed in and out of the center canal of the spine, nourishing your discs as you move. During the day, you lose fluid from the spine (especially when you sit). Think of a Slinky—when it's stretched open, it has space and length; when it contracts, it loses length, like the spine. Did you ever notice that you are shorter (by one and a half inches!) at the end of the day? Fluid loss is why. In the evening, you're more flexible, making injury less likely.

Don't settle for pain . . . ever.

My Posture

When I was growing up, my friends used to tease me: "Roberta, you idolize your mother." I never understood what they meant until later on in life. My mother always stood, sat, and walked with poise. I called my mother "Queen Jean" because she carried herself with majestic posture. She accepted her age with dignity, and always with wonderful posture.

My mother finally confessed that she went to the Barbizon School of Modeling and Etiquette. There she learned how to sit and stand properly, along with table manners, weight management, and overall poise. (If you want to psychoanalyze me, maybe that's why I subconsciously specialized in fantastic posture." The apple doesn't fall far from the tree.)

When I was studying at the Jacques Dalcroze School of Eurythmics in Brussels, Belgium, Patou, my teacher, once proclaimed, "Roberta, *tu marches comme un canard.*" Translation: "Roberta, you walk like a duck." Well, I thought I would die. Firstly, I had no idea. Secondly, I was mortified that she embarrassed me in front of my classmates.

My revenge, at age twenty-two: my lifelong study of how to sit, stand, and walk with good posture. My mean teacher was right. I led my walk head first as if I had to get somewhere quickly. When I looked in a mirror, reality struck. I really did walk with my head out like a duck. And it wasn't a pretty sight! My research is not over and never will be, because you can't coast on good posture. You must recreate good posture from moment to moment every single day.

Tip Sheet: Ten Ways to Improve Your Posture

1. Avoid sitting too long. Get up every hour and do posture stretches, then go back to what you're doing.
2. Avoid the postural pitfalls: sunken chest, rounded spine, hips thrust forward. Allow your neck to release, and balance your head forward and up; allow your back to lengthen and your shoulders to widen and expand. Loosen

the pelvis by dropping your buttocks down towards the heels.

3. Practice good posture every day. Habits of a lifetime cannot be changed in one day.

4. Use a mirror every day to reinforce good posture. Make sure head is over shoulders, shoulders over hips, and hips not too arched, not too tucked.

5. When you walk, let your legs and hips set the rhythm and speed. Do not try to walk faster by forcing the arms to set the pace or swinging them faster than the legs.

6. Make sure you walk, sit, and stand with good posture.

7. Lie on the floor completely stretched out to realign your body. Make sure both the right and left sides of your body are symmetrical. Rebalance your head, neck, shoulders, back, buttocks, thighs, calves, ankles, and feet.

8. Make sure your shoulders are always rolled back. Do a posture check by lifting the breastbone upward. Breathe deeply and fill the belly, ribs, and chest with air.

9. Fight gravity and stretch every joint and muscle every day. Stretching is like dessert. It gives you the sweet taste of working muscles: long, pliable, and ready for *action*!

10. Perform all activities with good use of the body. Work, playing with kids, doing household chores, sitting for long hours, traveling, playing an instrument, and sports can be done more easily and effortlessly with the correct use of your body.

IMPROVING POSTURE

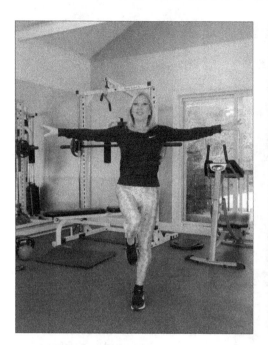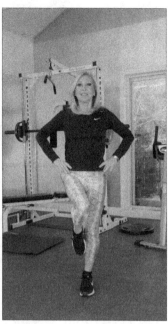

Proper Standing Posture.

Step 1. Bring your chin back, and bring your shoulders back and down. With arms outstretched, stand on one foot, and raise the other knee up. Balance in this position for a few seconds and change to other leg. (Hold on to stable surface, wall, or ballet barre if needed.)

Step 2. Same as previous exercise, with hands on hips.

For best posture, keep the lift in the breastbone, the back of the head lifted forward and upward. Use your full height while balancing on one leg at a time. Improves balance, posture, and alignment.

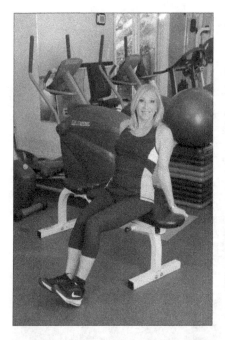

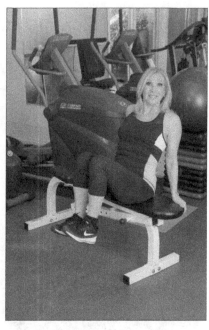

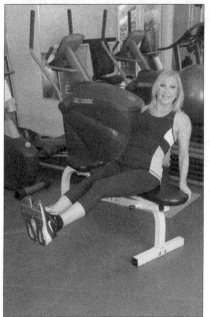

Proper Seated Posture Exercise

Step 1. Sit tall with breastbone lifted, hands toward back of seat. Roll the shoulders back and down, flex feet, and sit tall.

Step 2. Maintain same posture, and lift both thighs up toward chest to work core muscles.

Step 3. Maintain lifting knees, and extend lower legs to work core and quadriceps (the walking muscles). Repeat sequence several times.

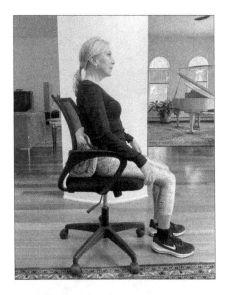

Proper Chair Posture

Roll up a towel or use a lumbar pillow and place it behind lower lumbar or middle back area. Pillow or towel can be placed vertically or horizontally. Experiment for comfort. Sit with hips against the back of chair, with thighs perpendicular to lower legs, feet flat on floor. Keep the breastbone lifted, the back of the head lifted forward and up. Roll shoulders back.

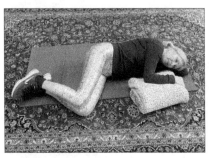

Lying posture

Lie on side with knees bent (fetal position). Place a pillow or rolled towel underneath elbow and forearm. Pillow can also be placed in between the knees for comfort. This position maintains the 3 natural curves of the spine.

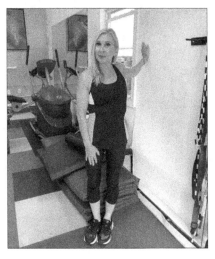

Posture, Balance, Alignment

Step 1. Stand with feet and ankles together. Place inside left-hand palm tight against wall to stretch the rotator cuff.

Step 2. Begin to walk away slowly from the raised arm until you feel a stretch inside the shoulder (rotator cuff) and chest (pectoral muscle). Repeat on the other side.

Chapter 4
Connecting the Mind, Body, and Back Pain

My body must be set a-going if my mind is going to work.
—Jean Jacques Rousseau

Diana, my childhood neighbor, helped shape my life's work. Diana was born deaf.

We communicated nonverbally. We read each others' lips and we "talked" on paper. Diana would come to my house and wait for me to finish practicing the piano. My mother was a strict disciplinarian and insisted that I finish homework and piano work before I played. Diana would sit patiently and watch me with great curiosity.

I decided that I would like to teach my friend to play the piano. I was fifteen at the time. My mother, as usual, gave me lots of encouragement. Not only did Diana learn how to play songs and memorize them, but she also corrected herself when she played a wrong note. She was sensing the vibrations in her fingers, her feet, and her whole body.

Diana made the mind-body connection early. She had a heightened awareness of all her senses to overcompensate for the hearing loss. For example, she was able to perceive outside noises like a car door slamming, a truck zooming by, the doorbell, or the telephone. All the sensations were internal for her. The sound waves were resonating through her body.

I was fascinated by her ability to sense sound and rhythm in the silence of her body. I put my philosophy on my bedroom wall: "If I can go through life and help just one person, I've accomplished enough for a lifetime." Diana attended Gallaudet University in Washington, D.C., a liberal arts university devoted to deaf people.

At the age of twenty, I spent my sophomore year in Jerusalem at Hebrew University. In addition to regular academic subjects, I had the good fortune to study at the Reuben Academy of Music. There I continued piano lessons and improvisational dance. I missed a lot of steps because I was not fluent in Hebrew. Since I didn't have the language facility, I had to rely on my body to receive the information.

The language was secondary to my urge to move with creativity and spontaneity. But eventually my Hebrew improved through the repetition of dance terminology. I discovered that dancing was a great tool for learning a foreign language.

During my year in Israel, I volunteered at the Blind Institute of Jerusalem. I taught dance movement therapy to blind children to help them communicate nonverbally and get in touch with their bodies. My teaching props were scarves. When the children waved them around, they were able to feel the motion and move with it. It gave the children a sense of balance and spatial awareness inherent to the mind-body connection. The fabrics gave definition to a wide range of physical sensations. These blind children made the connection by using their sense of touch, breath, and movement. My life's work had its beginnings there.

At age twenty-two, I married and moved to Brussels, Belgium. I studied at the Jacques Dalcroze School of Eurythmics. The Dalcroze method, which is taught internationally, was originally developed for children to coordinate musical rhythm with body movement.

Looking back, I giggle when I think of what I did each day. I remember shadow dancing on the wall; making my body into a sculpture of a swan, an eagle, or odd geometric shapes; jumping, skipping, hopping, and leaping in rhythm to the different beats and songs the teacher played on the piano. Once again, I was exploring the mind-body connection.

I submitted my application for a master of science program at Hunter College in New York City when I was living in Europe. In lieu of a personal interview, I sent a videotape of myself dancing.

I set up a studio in my neighbor's backyard in Brussels. I danced around the yard like a butterfly and any other animate or inanimate object I could conjure up in my imagination. That must have looked hilarious, since my neighbors, Sofie and Michel, stood at their window, laughing at the "*folle américaine.*" That "crazy American" was accepted into Hunter's Master of Science, Dance-Movement Therapy Program. As part of the education, we were trained to read people's body language and interpret it psychologically.

From that point on, my purpose in life became clear. I wanted to help people reach their full potential through the physical body.

While I was at Hunter College, I had a one-year internship with people with chronic schizophrenia at Creedmore Psychiatric Hospital, in Queens, New York. I used dance-movement therapy as the mode of communication. Although these people were extremely maladjusted and shut down, they still experienced emotions that they couldn't articulate verbally. The internship was an intense exerience for me as I saw patients releasing fears, depression, and other anxieties through movement.

The body's language is crystal clear. My mentor Don Gabor, a communication expert and author of *Speaking Your Mind in 101 Difficult Situations*, states: "Body language and non-verbal signals account for over 70 percent of all communication, voice tone and words are the remaining 30 percent. Body language influences how others feel and react when they talk to you."

Through forty years of teaching and researching, I have learned that making a silent connection between mind and body is the key to maintaining physical and emotional balance.

My purpose is to engage you in a process that will make you feel more in control of your back health. The connection between mind and body is the preliminary step to healing back pain. Once you are conscious of your physical body and you begin to notice your breath, you will become more sensitive to the kinks in your muscles. For example, you might feel tight in your upper back and loose in the middle section, with a shooting pain in your lower back. This is a sign that you have already become more sensitive to your back. And that is the mind-body connection!

The Inner Dialogue

Exploring with your senses gives you useful information about your mind and body. For example, the sense of smell can provoke memories, soothe the psyche, or stimulate pleasure. Touch can comfort you or make you uncomfortable. The sight of something beautiful can create loving thoughts; the sight of something ugly can make you angry.

Taste can be manipulated in hundreds of ways. Food can taste sweet, sour, bitter, spicy, or salty. Foods can alter your mood. In fact, many cultures use spices to make you feel calm, hyper, or serene. Spices are also used for medicinal purposes.

Hearing classical music can relax you. Rock music can charge you. Latin music can excite you. Dancing the tango cheek to cheek can bring out your deepest feelings of intimacy with your partner and your own body.

As you heighten your sensory awareness, you continue to expand the pleasures and possibilities your body can experience. You begin to connect your mind to your body.

Spending time in nature has many healing benefits. Watching the ocean waves, a calm lake, or a trickling stream is peaceful and calming. Studies show that simply looking at a body of water improves the mood. Hiking vigorously or walking in the woods can have meditative effects: the breath slows, the mind relaxes, and somehow physical and men-

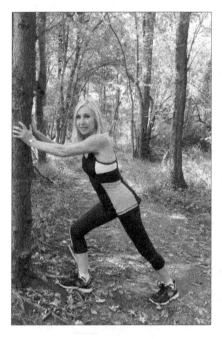
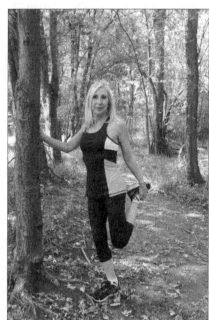

Step 1. Face a wall (or tree if outdoors); press hands flat against surface. Lunge forward with front leg, step straight back with other leg, and keep the heel down. This stretches the heel cord, Achilles tendon, and calf.

Step 2. Stand tall and bend the back leg up toward buttock while holding top of foot in hand to stretch the quadricep (front thigh).

Step 3. Go outdoors in nature and begin to breathe deeply, inhaling and exhaling slowly to calm your mind and body. This can be done seated, standing. or walking.

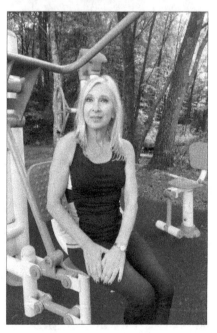

tal stress subsides. Noticing the trees and flowers and the beauty of the natural surroundings leads to a more positive outlook on your circumstances. Being outside in nature elicits the relaxation response and has a tranquilizing effect on the mind.

As you begin to experience life with all your senses, subtle messages will become clearer. If there is pain, you won't ignore it, hoping it will magically disappear. If you're tired, you'll rest. If you are hungry, you'll eat. If you want to trim down, you'll make the right choices. You will gain a deeper understanding of who you are and how you operate.

Babies process information through motor learning before their cognitive abilities develop. We are born communicating our needs nonverbally before we learn to speak. Babies are natural at crying out their physical needs. Adults, on the other hand, frequently ignore muscle and joint pain, hoping it will magically go away. My goal is to provide you with a positive outcome to reduce back pain.

The body doesn't lie.
—MARTHA GRAHAM

The Missing Link

Most people live from the neck up, never realizing that the rest of their body is ready, willing, and able to participate. Perhaps our goal-oriented work ethic forces us into fast-forward thinking. We plan the next step, the next thought, the next movement that is necessary for productivity.

But it is also imperative to prioritize the body. The body craves attention. The body's voice in overdrive sounds something like this: "Listen, listen, listen to me, and take one step at a time:" We need to slow down, if even for a megabyte, and take a pause and a deep breath. Just a simple step like this can create profound change and help you to relax your back. You may realize that it is no fun to be in pain and you have the tools to change it. Don't ignore your back pain. Exercise will bring you magical relief.

The Roman poet Juvenal was right in asserting that you should pray for a "strong body in a strong mind." Aristotle believed in the "cerebral satisfaction of exercise." Aristotle, who made a habit of walking while thinking or lecturing to his students, maintained that exercise made his mind more lucid. His students reported feeling more relaxed and disciplined, more self-confident and healthier-looking, and most importantly, having a stronger sense of being at one with themselves.

Your Body Is Your Guide
Locating Your Center

If you've ever taken dance or yoga classes, no doubt you've heard the teacher remind you to move from your center. It's a term that's used often. So what does *center* mean?

It's easiest to explain by doing the opposite. When you move your arm as an isolated body part, it's like an empty sleeve. It lacks energy and breath. It feels limp and appears lifeless.

Your center isn't an exact anatomical place, like your heart or your lungs. It is an area of energy located in your belly. You can place your hand over your belly and feel it. There is no mystery to finding your center. You can locate it by experimenting with movement and breath and feeling the acute differences in mental focus, energy, vitality, and peace of mind. You can catch glimpses of your center after a yoga class, tai chi, or meditation session. When you begin to move from your center, your whole body becomes well coordinated. Coordination is what happens when basketball players make a hoop. You can see the energy as they connect to the ball, the hoop, and their center.

It's hard to hold tension when your body is in harmony. It's easier to find that harmony, the stillness within. Centering affects every area of your life. Stick with me. I plan to lead you to your center.

Tai Chi: Chinese Martial Arts for Movement, Balance and Health

n the practice of tai chi, the energy center or belly area is called the *dantian*. Tai chi, like yoga, uses the breath through each movement. Tai chi is used as a path of inspiration and a guide to relaxation and health. Described as "moving meditation," tai chi has been used to counter depression, foster optimism and self-confidence, and unleash creativity.

Because it doesn't put stress on the joints, this discipline is perfect for the aging body. It improves balance and posture, which can be applied to every sport, including walking. Practicing tai chi teaches proper breathing techniques, promotes better coordination and posture, and creates a natural flow to movement patterns. You learn to move from your center.

Improve Your Body Awareness

Only you can hear what your body needs. But are you listening? For example, how often have you taken the time to simply *rest and do nothing?*

Body awareness gives you a greater sense of timing, energy, and action. Life is about balance, not perfection. Awareness teaches an understanding of the language of the body. Something as simple as dancing, hiking, biking, or massage can make you feel good.

Feeling good pays off twice. It directly improves biological functions as well as increasing feel-good alpha waves. When you feel good, you produce happy hormones, such as endorphins, epinephrine, dopamine, and seratonin, which produce a euphoric state.

Health Is a Choice

The Connection

Become conscious of any physical pain, tension, stress, or fatigue. Repeat how you are feeling over and over again until you hear your inner voice say, "I am anxious, my back hurts, I am completely exhausted, I am content."

Give yourself permission to rest and remove exhaustion from your body. Once you feel refreshed, exercise will energize you. Use your breath to connect to any movement you do, such as yoga, stretching, weight lifting, aerobics, walking, dancing, hiking, biking, swimming, or skiing.

Awareness Technique

Sensory Stretch

Purpose: to feel each part of your body in relation to the floor and to develop a kinesthetic awareness of your body in space. (*Kinesthetic* is derived from *kinesthesis*, which means the *sensory perception of movement*.)

Lie on your back with legs long and arms overhead. Stretch the right arm and the right leg out straight. Inhale as you stretch and exhale on the release. Repeat on the left side. Next, stretch both arms and legs. Arch your back; tense all the muscles while you inhale. Exhale, let go, and relax on the floor.

Ken Kerbs Back Exercise Routine

Ken Kerbs, photojournalist who's carried his cameras on his shoulders for decades, does these and other back and core exercises every morning, seven days a week!

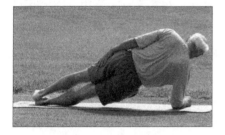

Side planks back

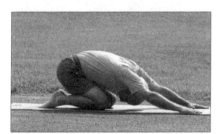

Stretch

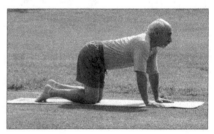

Cat

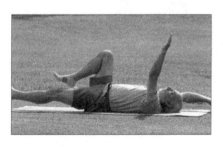

Leg lifts

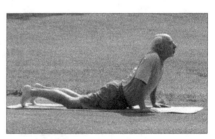

Upward dog

Chapter 5
Alternative Body Therapies for Reducing Back Pain

Movement is life; without movement, life is unthinkable.
—Moshe Feldenkrais

When I was growing up, my father and I had a stormy relationship. He'd say black, and I'd say white. What saved us was singing and dancing.

My father loved to hear me play the piano and sing Broadway show tunes. He taught me how to swing dance in our living room when I was in my teens. Dad's face lit up when we were dancing. It was the only time I could relax and express myself freely and still get approval. Looking back, I realize that singing and dancing were my way of surviving. Words were irrelevant. My feelings of anger, pain, frustration, and hopelessness seemed to fade into the background, replaced by happiness and joy.

The truth is that all forms of dance and movement can be healing physically as well as psychologically. Ballroom dancing, the tango, rumba, meringue, salsa, cha-cha, foxtrot, waltz, and swing dancing bring emotional release if you let go of your feelings and dance from your gut . . . with passion. Moving is magic!

Although there are dozens of body therapy methods, each one teaches focusing techniques for increased movement potential. All of these methods use touch, gentle rolling, energy infusion, hands-on manipulation, and/or floor movements. The movements are designed to improve health, correct alignment, decrease back and neck pain and tension, and ground the participant in the mind-body connection. Most notably, all body therapies are done slowly to help establish new patterns. Why? The body learns (or unlearns) slowly, but it never forgets.

For the past thirty plus years of working with "normal" people as a group exercise instructor and trainer, I've observed physical, mental, and emotional imbalances. I try to bridge those gaps. I strive to give my clients a deeper experience of thinking, feeling, sensing, and moving the body. I use a variety of disciplines, including movement therapy, dance, yoga, the Alexander Technique, the Feldenkrais Method, and traditional exercise. The goal: to rebalance the body to a pain-free state.

I firmly believe that exercise done solely for the purpose of looking good is only part of the picture. Long lasting changes happen when you slow down and deepen your mind/body connection. I admit, I always have a hard time adjusting to slow results, let alone moving slowly. If it wasn't jazz dance, it was boring. The thought of a yoga class was out of the question until one of my former boyfriends invited me to join him in one. I became hooked. I have learned that my black-and-white view of the world prevented me from staying open to new possibilities, physically and emotionally.

Face it: we are all hooked on quick and instant results. Change is frightening on many levels. My yoga boyfriend once told me to "be a human being, not a human doing." The "being" part was the challenge for me, as it is for many people.

The body holds truths, secrets, lies, distortions, deep pain, unreleased emotion, and frozen feelings, which translate into psychological tension as well as physical limitation.

As my business grew, I began to explore many other body movement therapies. Although my intention was to gather information for my clients, I realized that I was going through a transformation of my own during this process. I was clear that I wanted to work with people in a more therapeutic, hands-on way.

Our bodies hold the key to what we need. This sensibility begins in infancy. But as we become adults, we are taught to repress our body's natural tendencies toward freedom of movement. We are taught to sit like a lady, stand up straight, and keep our hands at our sides and off our laps. This is hardly the breeding ground for easy, natural movement.

Body therapy methods include Feldenkrais, Alexander, bioenergetics, yoga, meditation, therapeutic touch, massage, myofascial release, Rolfing, reiki, and tai chi. Even ballroom dancing can bring you back to your center. Back to where we were as children . . . moving freely without restriction.

> *When you lie down and are quiet, you can*
> *feel the fact that your body is never still.*
> —ELAINE SUMMERS, BODY THERAPIST

Body Awareness

The ideal body functions without strain on the muscles or joints: it is a body that moves freely. The antithesis is the body racked with ongoing muscle tension, resulting in major postural imbalances. Common physical manifestations of habitual tension include hyperextended cervical (neck) and lumbar (low back) curves, raised and rounded shoulders, locked and knocked knees, and pronated (inwardly rotated) feet. Be aware if you are suffering from these problems and talk to your doctor.

Body awareness teaches an understanding of the language of the body. A person may be saying one thing, but the body another. Moshe Feldenkrais asserts that poor movement patterns often come from not understanding how to coordinate your body in motion. Many theorists also conclude that emotional attitudes are often connected to muscular tensions.

Muscle tension distorts awareness by perpetuating a tense pattern which feels normal but isn't. Changing a dysfunctional pattern can be very uncomfortable. It takes concentration and awareness to reestablish communication between the muscles and the brain.

But the proof is there. F.M. Alexander, founder of the Alexander Technique, learned to reshape habits that were causing his voice loss. Elsa Gindler, a body therapist, cured her tuberculosis by teaching herself to breathe only with her healthy lung, letting the diseased lung rest.

The mind-body connection is inherent to the nature of body therapies. The specific use of movement differs with each method, yet they share common goals, including release of muscular tension, reduction of effort during movement, increase in range of motion and flexibility, improved coordination, increased physical awareness, and enhanced body image. Reported changes in attitudes and emotions include reduction of anxiety, a feeling of "being in the present," greater openness to new ideas and experience, greater ability to solve problems, a more tolerant view of others, and a greater sense of well-being and positive self-esteem.

The body must be treated as a whole if real integration is to occur. Your physical body is your own creation, produced from a lifetime of experiences and habits. For the body to sustain change, the emotional and attitudinal postures that formed it in the first place must also be changed. Muscular movement without consciousness doesn't seem to last. I've seen many people work out day in and day out without ever really changing their bodies. Eating habits did not change, weight did not change, body image did not change, posture did not change, and confidence and self-esteem weren't significantly changed.

The greatest changes in the physical body occur when there are changes in awareness and attitude. For example, if you have a "new" body through weight loss, you will most likely feel different. A changed self-image comes only with alterations including a new belief system. This occurs through the process of the body "speaking to the mind."

These human potential techniques teach you to see yourself from many angles, viewpoints, and perspectives. You place yourself in a position of greater honesty and intimacy. A fully developed self means that you approach mastery of self-awareness and body awareness.

But remember that it's an ongoing journey that ebbs and flows like the tides. You may feel like exploring more at certain times in your life than at others.

We all need a break from intense personal exploration to simply enjoy life. If you are in a period of emotional turmoil, it is not a display of weakness to seek help, nor is it a shameful act. In fact, it's a sign of willingness to face the truth and recover from conflict. Many people choose verbal psychotherapy as the sole means of therapy. The mind-body route is a holistic approach to the physical, emotional, and spiritual being.

There are many body therapies, but they lead to the same road. Find your own path. I am outlining a few methods that have been my path toward personal transformation: kinesthetic awareness, myofascial release, the Feldenkrais Method, the Alexander Technique, and yoga.

Kinesthetic Awareness

Have you ever heard that most people only use 10 percent of their brainpower? Would it surprise you to learn that you only use a minuscule portion of your total body in all areas of your life, including daily chores, athletic activities, and work tasks? Compare yourself to a Balanchine dancer. The muscular effort required to kick your leg high, stand on your toes with perfect balance, and use one body part while stilling the rest of your body takes an acute awareness. This is called the sixth sense—the kinesthetic sense. Kinesthetic awareness requires developing the physical sensation of movement in each and every muscle and bone in your body.

Body therapist Elaine Summers developed the method known as Kinetic Awareness to help people connect to their bodies. It uses a ball to stretch and massage the neck and back of the head. You lie on the floor, rotating your head slowly on a small, spongy ball to release tensions. Elaine believes that this is the way to finding your dynamic center.

Myofascial Release

The good news: *muscles don't know age.* Everybody can return to a good flexibility level. Why? Connective tissue is made of collagen, a protein substance. As you age, collagen becomes like tight threads in your body, keeping your muscles from moving freely. Staying flexible keeps collagen from mounting and thereby restricting movement.

The fascia is the outer layer of muscle. It acts as a shock absorber and has the strength of a radial tire. Think of the fascia system like layers of an onion. The fascia tightens, and slowly over time we tighten, tighten, and tighten. The fascia wraps around the belly of the muscle like a rope. Finally, it loses its fluid content and crystallizes into those knots we get.

Tight fascia affects the digestive, respiratory, and circulatory functions as well as the musculoskeletal system. Spontaneity of motion is lost, and pain occurs. The slightest motion throws you out of function. We commonly see the results of tight fascia in old age, but also in very athletic people who have done lots of strength training but have neglected stretching. Stooped posture, rigidity, hip imbalances, shoulder blade unevenness, one shoulder higher than the other, leg length discrepancy, and frozen facial expressions are characteristic of tight fascia.

When fascia is released, elimination, breathing, and circulation improve. When the myofascial system works well, you move gracefully and spontaneously.

Myofascial Release is a medical therapy that helps to correct myofascial tension. Physical therapist John Barnes, president of the Myofascial Release Treatment Centers in Paoli, Pennsylvania, and Sedona, Arizona, made this method world-renowned. Over the years he has trained 20,000 physical therapists and health care professionals to use these techniques, which include a specific kind of deep tissue massage that helps unlock the fascia that have crystallized into killer knots.

Myofascial release feels like a good stretch. Combined with regular stretching, it guarantees a more flexible, younger-looking, pain-free body. It seems like a small price to pay for such great relief.

The Feldenkrais Method

Moshe Feldenkrais (1904–84) has been a major force in movement awareness. An Israeli, Feldenkrais was a physicist and engineer as well as a black belt in judo. His discoveries came about as a result of knee injuries he suffered from soccer in his teens. When surgery was the recommended course for treatment (with a 50 percent chance of successful recovery), Feldenkrais decided to take his own path. Through his knowledge of anatomy, physiology, engineering, and physics, he developed the Feldenkrais Method. He worked miracles with people who had minor muscular problems as well as disabling muscle spasms, strokes, cerebral palsy, multiple sclerosis, and arthritis.

Feldenkrais's philosophy about movement encompasses walking, sitting, and lying. He professed that you should be able to move in any direction with ease. This method involves two types of movement lessons. In a group setting, they are known as Awareness Through Movement (ATM). These group lessons enable you to participate on your own with verbal directives from a Feldenkrais practitioner. Individual sessions are known as Functional Integration. These one-on one, hands-on sessions involve touch and gentle manipulation. You are fully clothed.

The teacher is your guide. According to New York City Feldenkrais practitioner John Link, "instructions are given verbally. Since the teacher doesn't demonstrate, their focus is on the student. The point is to encourage the student to pay attention to their own movement rather than imposing any external standards about how the movement should be done. The longer you do this, the simpler your movements become, the more you do just what's essential to carry out your intention. The lesson belongs to you. Unlike fitness classes or one-on-one training, the teacher doesn't impose their own agenda."

The premise behind Feldenkrais is that almost any human activity involves movement in more than one joint. For example, when you lift a fork to your lips, there is movement in many parts of your upper body. The Feldenkrais technique teaches one to make light, easy, and graceful movements by integrating muscle efforts. The most efficient movements use smaller, weaker muscles to deal with fine adjustments, leaving bigger movements to larger and stronger muscles.

In order to become a Feldenkrais practitioner, you have to go through a four-year training program that takes place in the summers. After two years of training, you become qualified to teach Awareness Through Movement lessons. After completing the full four years, you are qualified to conduct Functional Integration lessons as well.

I am not a Feldenkrais practitioner. However, after seventeen years of studying the method, I recognize its magnificent benefits in mobility, back and neck pain relief, more coordinated movement, and overall mind-body integration. I encourage all my clients to use the method for a variety of reasons, including a pain-free back.

After each Awareness Through Movement lesson, I'm always amazed at how sensitive you become to the discrepancies between the right and left sides of your body. The method enables you to access every inch of your back.

The technique also enables you to feel more grounded, centered, and self-defined. Lessons involving breathing changes will leave you feeling liberated and relaxed. Through the Feldenkrais experience, you may experience smoother and more rhythmic movement.

Exercises based upon the Feldenkrais Method

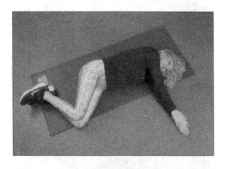

Step 1. Lie in a fetal position. Keep upper arm and hand on top of lower arm and hand.

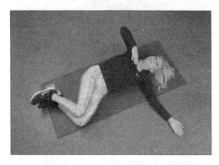

Step 2. Glide the upper arm slowly across the chest, maintaining contact with the lower arm, then with the chest, until arm is outstretched on the floor.

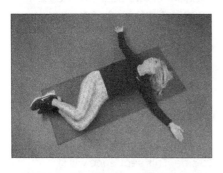

Step 3. Slowly turn head to look at the outstretched arm.

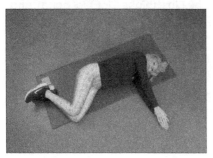

Step 4. Return upper arm to position of departure. This "body harp" sequence will increase mobility in the spine to ease movement. It will relax the back and neck.

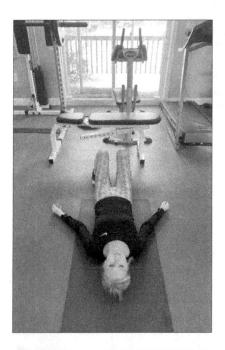

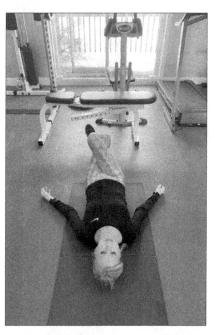

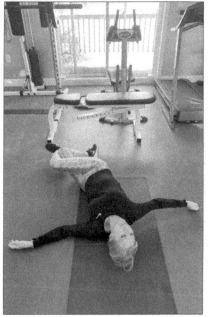

Step 1. Lie on a mat on the floor, with lower back pressed into the mat, shoulders back and down, knees hip distance apart, arms outstretched away from the sides of the body.

Step 2. Cross one leg over the other.

Step 3. With outstretched arms, drop both legs to one side slowly, breathe in through the nose, then exhale slowly. Repeat sequence on other side, continuing from side to side. This sequence will stretch the hips, thighs (iliotibial band), and spine. It loosens the entire torso and lower back.

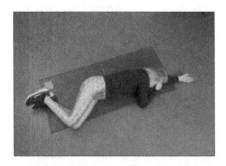

Step 1. Lie in fetal position, with palm of hand pressed firmly on forehead. Keep hand on forehead the entire time.

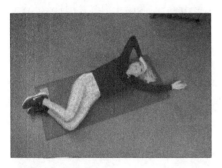

Step 2. Gently lift the elbow toward the ceiling while moving the head slowly to the opposite side.

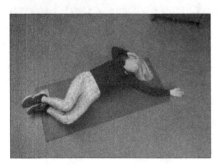

Step 3. Stretch the elbow as far back toward floor as possible in order to approach the floor on opposite side. Move slowly to gauge how far you are able to move before you feel pain. Return to the original position. This relaxes the neck muscles (cervical spine), decreases neck pain, and improves mobility. Repeat sequence a few times.

In a one-on-one Functional Integration lesson, John Link asked me what I'd like to work on. Since I had no particular pain, I suggested we work on my age-old issue of body image and weight, which has plagued me since I was thirteen years old.

At the beginning of the lesson, John asked me to lie back on a padded table with my legs extended. He proceeded to guide me through various movements, such as rolling my head left and right and rolling my legs in and out.

John asked me to pay attention. As he moved my limbs gently, I noticed that my breathing pattern changed. After an hour of being gently manipulated, I felt as if I'd had a great massage. At the end of the session, I felt extremely focused and more self-assured. I experienced the body-mind connection. Whenever I feel out of sorts, unbalanced, upset, or confused, I take a Feldenkrais lesson to bring me back to who I really am.

According to Marci Lindheimer, founder of The Feldenkrais Leaming Center in New York City, "The Feldenkrais Method is an educational modality, not a medical one. It's a neuromuscular exchange. . . . the movements are a means to work with the brain. The movement provides new information to the neuromuscular system enabling change in one's organization and gravity which enhances efficiency, coordination and ease of movement."

Lindheimer notes that as we age, we tend to repeat our habits and prefer certain movement patterns, so we don't get the full gamut of movement. That's why people become more stooped or tilted to one side. The object of Feldenkrais lessons is to explore more movement options on a regular basis to access more spontaneous movement.

The Feldenkrais Method caters to the rhythm of your own body. What a concept! Your movement, like your thumbprint, is different from that of every other person in the world. Most of us fitness enthusiasts are brainwashed to believe that the only way to change your body is to push it to its limits and force it to do what is unnatural. Good news! You don't have to live that way all the time. The Feldenkrais Method gives you permission to be exactly where you are with your body in the present moment. For instance, aren't there days when you're in slow motion, where you don't feel like competing, lifting heavy weights, or running on the treadmill? Those are days when the Feldenkrais method would be beneficial, and you still feel you're using your body. The brain absorbs gentle and comfortable movements. By contrast, strenuous movement leads the brain to protect the body from pain and thus hinders the learning of new information. With Feldenkrais lessons, posture and gait improve, and the hips and ribs loosen and have greater freedom. New patterns of movement become imprinted on your nervous system. For instance, you automatically begin to incorporate your back, ribs, and pelvis, not just your hands and wrists, when you work at the computer. In all areas of life, you learn to move from the center of your body. It's a way to feel more at home in your body.

This method can be used for a variety of reasons and executed either on the floor or in a chair. Let's say your shoulder hurts you, and you're used to lifting heavy weights: thirty-, forty-, fifty-pound dumbbells or more. While you lift the weight, you probably don't detect where the pain originates or how you're using your arms or shoulders to contribute to it. Reducing the weights down to the lightest featherweight, let's say five or ten pounds allows you to contact the origin of the pain. Only then can you discover other movement options and avoid pain.

The same theory can be applied to lifting kids, groceries, or laundry. By taking movement down to the slowest, lightest, easiest common denominator, you will learn to move more comfortably.

Hey, all of you stretch-averse guys, take note! The Feldenkrais Method teaches you how to stretch within a comfortable range while avoiding pain. Case in point: one of my clients, a strapping six-foot, four-inch guy, was in brutal back and neck pain. I kept him off weights and on Feldenkrais for six weeks. Today he is back to lifting heavy weights without pain.

When movement is not well organized, there is no grace. The longer you do this method, the more graceful you become. You acquire an ease of movement.

I'll never forget one of my first private ballroom dance lessons with my husband. He was so busy learning the steps that he forgot that I was dancing with him, and he forcefully threw me over his foot. He tripped me accidentally (I think), and I went flying across the floor and fell flat on my belly. That wasn't the sad part. The sad part was that he didn't even notice that I was gone. He kept on dancing! SOS! (P.S. After thirteen years of lessons, my husband became a wonderful ballroom dance partner.)

Although, as I have mentioned, I am not a certified Feldenkrais practitioner, I have combined seventeen years of Feldenkrais training, my position as a dance/movement therapist, and over 200 hours of back care education through the American Back Society and developed my own body formula. Over a twelve-year period working at the Williams Island Spa in Aventura, Florida, I carefully choreographed a series of exercises for people with back, neck, shoulder, hip, and knee pain.

My students at the spa were extremely pleased with the results of this soft movement and showed remarkable improvements. They practiced some of the lessons on their own, which was beneficial to their healing.

Aggressive back rehab is most effective with the Feldenkrais Method. Movements are done gently on the floor under the supervision of a trained Feldenkrais practitioner.

You can't control the waves, but you can learn how to surf.
—YOGI MASTER

Yoga: The Peace Potential

Yoga has become the buzzword for exercise in the new millennium. We overstrained, overaerobicized, and overstepped the eighties. The nineties were about stretching, alignment, and spirituality. And people are getting hooked on the high from the feeling of deep peace that yoga brings. Yoga means unity!

Yoga, a practice that is 4,000 years old, makes the body appear younger and stretches the back. I was introduced to a yoga teacher a few years ago. His body was that of a lithe, agile, swift, thirty-year-old. If I hadn't seen his face and hair, I wouldn't have known he was seventy. With regular practice, yoga can interrupt and even reverse the biomarkers of the aging body: stiff, stooped, achy, and arthritic.

I started studying yoga when my then-boyfriend took me to the World Yoga Center in New York City. The class was held in a simple room with a wooden floor, some mats, and no mirrors.

At my first class, I was my usual agitated and hyper self, thinking about what I had to do when the class was over. Everyone was asked to lie in the relaxation posture, flat on the back, with legs extended. The teacher's voice was low yet strong, soft but clear, quiet yet penetrating. I'd never heard a voice like that before. Her voice led my mind to be silent, and I began to listen attentively to her directions: breathe deeply, quiet your mind, be still. Her voice enabled me to lose self-consciousness and focus on her words. I was able to let go of my mental lists and step into a new space . . . a sacred space.

The yoga postures were challenging, but nothing I couldn't handle with all the dance classes Id taken. For me, the postures were peripheral to the serenity I was experiencing. Even though the class was two hours long, I had gone from type A to Zen. I felt relaxed, calm inside, centered and focused.

I continued to go back to this class week after week, and it has become my retreat. I do yoga especially in times of emotional turmoil. The tightness in my throat and chest open, and I feel solace. Yoga is therapeutic. It transforms energy and makes your body tingle. It doesn't change reality but helps you deal with the circumstances in your life calmly . . . or at least more calmly than otherwise.

There are many forms of yoga (see below). They all involve deep breathing and postures known as *asanas*, which provide deep stretching, alignment, power, and flexibility. Combining the postures with deep breathing and relaxation releases the healing and regenerative forces within yourself. Sessions usually end with a period of meditation to help absorb the aftereffects of the asanas. Yoga has been said to relieve minor ailments including insomnia, muscle pain, old injuries, premenstrual syndrome (PMS), and back or neck aches.

Yoga is also known as the body work for meditators. The postures make the back flexible and strong in order to tolerate sitting in the upright meditation posture.

Base your yoga practice on the pleasure principle: if it hurts, it's not good for you, and if it feels good, it is good for you. Trust yourself! One precaution for anyone with back or neck pain: don't do any posture that exacerbates pain. Some postures prolong forward flexion (bending), thus straining the lumbar muscles. Other postures prolong a back extension (bending), which may increase pain. Stay within your comfort zone, even if a teacher is encouraging you to stretch beyond your means. Listen to your body first, your teacher second. Always!

Following is a brief roundup of a few basic kinds of yoga training:

Ashtanga yoga is often called "Power Yoga." It brings alignment to the body, eases pain and tension, and releases stress, toxins and tightness from the body-mind. It is exhilarating and restorative.

Hatha yoga is the ancient science of physical, mental, and spiritual well-being. You learn how to examine, control, and use your breath to relieve body-mind tension. Instead of having opposing sets of muscles fighting each other, you teach your muscles to trust one another and work in sync. Each class is structured to ensure a balanced workout of all muscles of the body. The session ends with a deep guided relaxation to release any remaining tension and promote a calm sense of well-being.

Integral yoga involves breathing, postures, chants, and mantras. A mantra is a subtle sound used to create a peaceful vibration and a feeling of well-being.

Iyengar yoga emphasizes the balance between strength, flexibility, and endurance. The practice develops self-awareness through precision in movement and attention to the more subtle aspects of posture and breath.

Kundalini yoga is very vigorous and uses the "breath of fire" technique to charge you up and "ignite the fires of energy in the body." Breathing is done with sealed lips and short breaths exhaled through the nostrils. The Sanskrit word *kundalini* means *coiled up like a spring.* The purpose of this type of yoga is to release untapped power within each of us.

Kripalu yoga is often referred to as the "yoga of consciousness." The focus is on integration of movement, breath, and awareness. This encourages a more deeply internal experience.

Restorative yoga is all about slowing down and opening your body through passive stretching. During the long holds of restorative yoga postures, your muscles relax deeply. It's a unique feeling because props such as bolsters (long pillows), blankets, and blocks are used to support your body. It reduces physical, mental, and emotional stress.

Every time you do yoga, you meet yourself. Your true nature emerges like mist rising from a lake. Yoga practice leads you to this clarity of mind, body, and spirit. That's enough of an incentive, isn't it?

The health benefits of yoga include decreased stress and tension, joint pain reduction, improved posture, expanded lung capacity (up to 40 percent), and decreased injury (due to greater flexibility). Most importantly—yoga is fun! Many avid runners, dedicated weight lifters, devoted tennis players, and golfers place yoga as their number one priority in workouts.

Yoga is the only form of exercise that keeps you balanced and centered without fail. If you feel listless and lifeless after you've worked out, something is wrong. You may be depleting your energy supplies rather than accessing energy. Your exercise routine may have become a little stale and in need of change. Ideally, you should feel full of pep after a workout. So, take a break from your killer routines and try the path of least resistance. Yoga will refresh, revitalize, and relax you every time.

Yoga is also a philosophy. It preaches simplicity, acceptance, peacefulness, and love. It's a wonderful way to balance a fast-paced and pressure-filled life. Furthermore, yoga teachers claim that practitioners are biologically seven years younger than people who don't practice. *Yoga is a lifestyle.*

Chapter 6
Back Pain and Breathing

Stress can change physiology and blood pressure. It can also cause neck and back pain, allergies, ulcers, anxiety and panic attacks, heart attacks, stroke, arrhythmia, chronic fatigue, stomach conditions, and eating disorders. The body's response to stress can cause mental fatigue and/or physical exhaustion. Stress does not magically go away. It is important to identify individual patterns of stress and learn to respond with the strategies listed below.

If your back pain is stress-related, you can learn to turn it off by creating a sacred space to experience deep states of calmness, centering, and stability. This space can be a quiet room to sit and think or meditate.

There are two ways of moving through stress—active and passive. You can burn it off in a gym. Active stress reduction includes cardiovascular exercise and weight lifting, for example. Passive stress reduction includes yoga, stretching, tai chi, meditation, and naps. Making time for yourself on a regular basis is key to stress management. Both active and passive methods will lead to positive thinking and improved mental focus. Exercise and meditation are both potent stress-relieving activities for everyday life. They are not mutually exclusive and can be done separately.

All about Breathing

Let's stop for a second. Take a moment to pause, shift your time dimension, and slow down. Breathe. You have more control over situations than you realize. Breathing—simply allowing air to come in and out of your body—is everything. The breath lifts the body, spirit, and energy. We can learn to use breathing rhythms to deepen the silent partners known as mind and body. Focus on the breath and stay present in the moment, not stuck in the past or worried about the future. This thinking can help access energy and free your mind.

Breathing and Relaxation Posture

Purpose: to calm the nervous system and experience inner peace.

Lie flat on your back with legs long and arms resting at your side. Slow your breathing down. Inhale deep cleansing energy; exhale to release fatigue and anxiety. Breathe a sigh of relief.

360-Degree Breaths

Place your hands on your waist, and notice the breath expand into your hands as you inhale (like an accordion opening). Feel the waist shrink as you exhale. Inhale slowly and exhale deeply.

Fill your belly like a balloon as you inhale, feel the air escaping as you exhale.

Fill the front, sides, and back of your ribs as you inhale; relax the ribs as you exhale.

Repeat this with your hands criss-crossed over your shoulders to feel your shoulders rise as you inhale and fall as you exhale.

Place your hands over your chest. Next, fill your chest as you inhale; relax the chest as you exhale. Let the breath out S-L-O-W-L-Y. You will expand through the chest as you inhale and contract the chest to exhale.

The Silent Posture

Purpose: to relieve stress, relax your mind, and balance your thoughts.

Sit in an easy cross-legged position, with your back upright propped against a wall or chair.

Exaggerate your breath. Begin to breathe deeply and slowly. As you inhale, count to 4; as you exhale, count to 8. Ignore outside distractions, and turn your consciousness within. Become a witness to your experience, not a participant. Sit in silence as long as you feel comfortable. This is a form of meditation, and it brings a sense of calmness and peace of mind.

Body Scan

Purpose: to become more intimately connected to each part of your body, to view your body objectively, and to experience it as an integrated unit. Keep your eyes closed to increase awareness of each part of your body.

Lie on your back in the relaxation posture. Begin to breathe deeply and exhale slowly. If your back or neck hurts, place a pillow or rolled-up towel underneath the backs of your knees and/or under your neck.

Notice the width and shape of your thighs as you inhale. As you exhale, consciously let go of your thighs.

Pay attention to one body part at a time. Begin with your toes. As you inhale, notice your toes, and as you exhale, release the toes from your awareness. As you inhale, notice your calves—their size, shape, and length. As you exhale, let your calves disappear from your mind.

Become aware of your belly as you inhale; pay attention to its roundness or flatness. Let your belly dissolve from your attention as you exhale.

Notice your chest and back as you inhale. Feel your back in contact with the floor. Then release the image from your mind as you slowly exhale.

Breathe in and visualize your arms: the length and width of your arms, hands, wrists, fingers, and every fingertip. Release tension from your arms, and let them sink into the floor as you exhale.

Breathe in and notice the details of your face. See your eyes, nose, cheeks, chin, ears, and hair. Relax your forehead and the lines of worry from your brow. Feel the release of the eyes, the jaw, the forehead. As you exhale, release the image of your face from your mind.

Inhale and visualize your entire body. Trace your silhouette with your mind. Exhale slowly, and allow your body's image to disappear. Enjoy this feeling of relaxation, and allow it to soothe you, comfort you, and wash the stress out of your mind and body.

The above breathing and relaxation techniques provide useful coping mechanisms. They won't eradicate problems but help create a sense of control over stress. Practice any of the various breathing techniques throughout the day. When you feel stressed, take a few minutes for yourself and simply inhale through the nose and exhale through pursed lips (eyes open or closed).

Nighttime is the perfect time to practice breathing. It's a soothing way to help you unwind and relax.

Five Ways to Improve Self-Care and Well-Being

1. Maintain a regular routine of back exercise.
2. Do a body scan, and check when you feel tension build up.
3. Do relaxation techniques to decrease muscular tension and enhance the breathing process.
4. Exercise a positive attitude and choose not to allow stress to get the best of you.
5. Breathe deeply to release pent-up tension and stress throughout the day.

Chapter 7
Sports, Exercise, and Back Pain

———•———

Sports and exercise both involve physical performance. Each requires flexible back muscles for maximum agility and strong abs (core muscles) to protect the back. The greater the trunk control, the greater the performance. Sports and exercise are exciting, spine-tingling, and fun! Yet these two of life's greatest pleasures cannot be fully enjoyed if you can't move freely.

"When your back is out, your brain is continuously firing without stopping. You can't think about anything else. You can't learn anything new," says Feldenkrais practitioner Marci Lindheimer. The last thing you can think about is getting out your golf clubs or taking a challenging exercise class. Even the thought of sitting at your desk or lifting your child can provoke anxiety. The back doesn't distinguish between activities. It simply registers pain.

The trunk is your base of power. The back, abdominal, hip, and leg muscles should merge to form this "girdle of strength." A strong trunk can defend you from back pain. Strong core muscles are key: they insulate the back. Even the impact of swinging a bat, golf club, or tennis racket can herniate a disc if you're not in shape. Often elbow, shoulder, and arm pain is a direct result of abdominal weakness.

Gain the Core Advantage!

The inner unit of the core musculature includes the diaphragm, iliocostalis, and transverse abdominis muscles. One of the most effective ways to train the inner core is to consciously brace the core while doing other exercises that require higher stability. Be aware of keeping your core stable as you execute any movement. To locate your core muscles, lie on the floor with legs extended and imprint the spine on the floor: press the spine downward into the floor, initiating the movement from the core muscles. The diaphragm functions with the abdominal muscles and pelvic floor to provide core stability when braced. A strong core will help you in all athletic endeavors as well as daily activities such as walking, reaching, lifting, twisting, and bending forward. A strong core synchronizes with the back to maintain a balanced, pain-free torso. Strengthening the back only is not enough to maintain a strong torso. It requires getting on a mat on the floor and working hard by focusing on pulling your belly button in toward the spine, then pressing the spine downward into the mat.

The perfect place to strengthen your core musculature is in a Pilates mat class. The instructors are extremely skilled and knowledgeable about developing core strength. Most gyms provide Pilates mat classes, which is much easier than doing it on your own. If anything is too difficult in a class because of back pain or weakness in your trunk, take it upon yourself to limit the intensity of the exercise. Only you know how your back feels.

In the words of veteran football player Sean Landeta, *"injuries and pro sports are like peanut butter and jelly. They go hand in hand. Almost every player in the NFL has a back problem."* Athletes need to become skilled at more than their sport. It's a known fact that balance, alignment, coordination, and cardiovascular conditioning improve performance. So do a strong core and back.

In the Gym

Certain exercise classes are contraindicated when you have back pain. In fact, the American College of Sports Medicine (ACSM) maintains that jumping or twisting with back or neck pain is unsafe. Running and high-impact jumping are out. My advice is to maintain proper posture during all exercise classes, and listen to your body first. If your teacher is doing something that doesn't feel right for your body, don't do it. Always cool down and stretch after class to reduce the possibility of injury.

Avoid step classes and high-impact aerobics if you have back pain. They put too much pressure on the lumbar discs.

Core Exercises

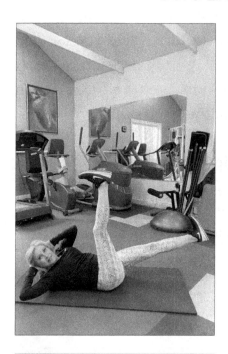
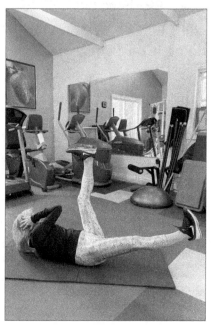

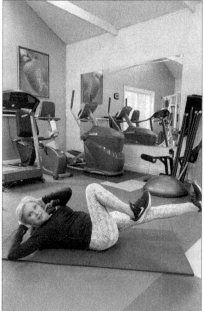

Step 1. Place hands behind the head. Lift one leg up straight toward ceiling, keeping other leg 3 inches off floor. Scissor the legs, alternating left and right sides (above left).

Step 2. Bring opposite elbow toward the opposite knee while scissoring legs to strengthen core muscles (above).

Step 3. Place hands behind the head. Bend one knee toward chest while extending other leg straight out (3 inches off the floor). Bring opposite elbow toward opposite knee (left). Then alternate sides. Repeat sequence 12 times.

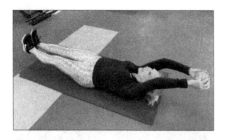

Step 1. Hold a light weighted ball or a softball. Lie on back; lift legs 3 inches off the floor. Reach the ball overhead with arms straight back overhead.

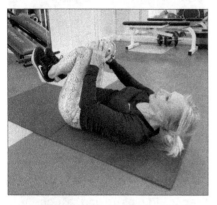

Step 2. Bend both knees in toward chest, reaching the ball toward the knees.

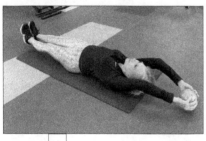

Step 3. Reach arms straight back and overhead again.

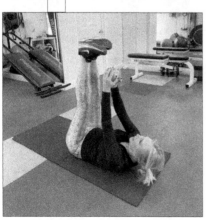

Step 4. Lift both legs straight up toward ceiling, and reach ball up toward toes. This is a 4-part sequence. Repeat entire sequence 4–8 times to strengthen core muscles. This can also be done without using a ball.

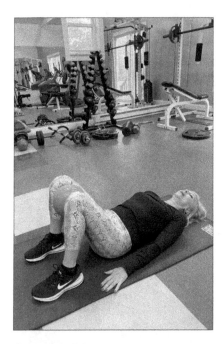 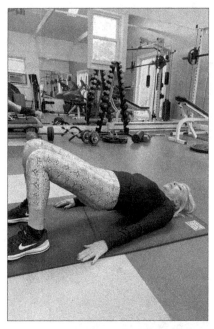

Step 1. Lie flat on your back with knees bent, feet flat on floor. Place a softball in between the knees. Tilt the pelvis under by pressing the lower back into the mat. Bring shoulders back and down. Squeeze the ball with the knees. This decreases the arch in the lower back.

Step 2. Lift hips up and rest on shoulders. Continue to squeeze the ball between knees. Then lower down in a controlled manner—upper back first, then middle back and lower back, down to floor last, undulating the spine. This sequence will help reverse postural lordosis.

Low or nonimpact aerobics are a better choice. Walking is the best option, both on land and in the water. Walking in water is easier on the joints than walking on land. Avoid conditioning classes that use heavy weights, as they will only exacerbate the pain. Using light weights (one to five pounds) should not be problematic. You can also take a break from weights altogether until you're back on track.

Nautilus equipment is a shoo-in for back pain if not used properly. Be careful not to arch the back while seated on a piece of equipment. The first step is to keep your lower back against the back of the seat. Again, brace your core muscles to properly place your back before using the required muscles to work the equipment. Try to keep the back of your head against the equipment for proper form, with chin tucked slightly to chest. If there is no back, place yourself in the pelvic tilt position, with a straight spine and lifted abdominals. Use your core muscles (not just your arms) to help lift, push, or press against the resistance. Connect your breath to the movement. Exhale as you exert effort; inhale as you release the weight.

Paulo Pinheiro is a personal trainer and owner of Exercise Excellence, a personal training studio in Tucson, Arizona. Notice the definition in Paulo's back muscles (next page). Even if you never achieve that level of back strength, practicing and reinforcing the exercises that develop these muscles will improve your current back condition. The key is consistency and discipline. Twice per week should bring results in four to six weeks.

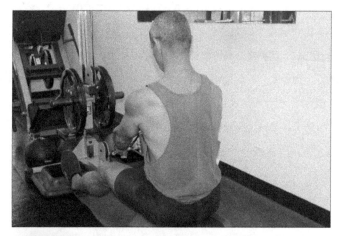

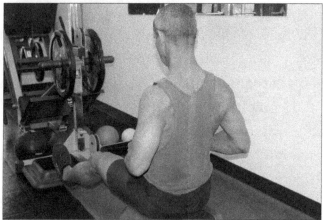

Cable Rower

Step 1. Sit with good posture. Bring shoulders back and down, chin back, and hold the position. Bend the knees to reach forward to hold handles of rower.

Step 2. Pull elbows back while squeezing shoulder blades together as the legs straighten, and bend to row. Repeat sequence 1 to 2 minutes. This tones and strengthens the middle back (rhomboids) and secondarily the latissimus dorsi and biceps.

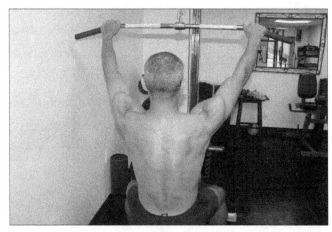

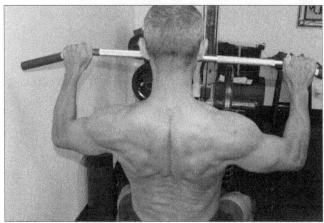

Lat Pulldown

Make sure the weight is comfortable, not too difficult to start, and not too light. Gradually add weight over time as you progress. It's always wise to get advice from a personal fitness trainer.

Step 1. Sit with good posture, chin back, breastbone lifted. Reach arms up to grab the handles of the bar wide out.

Step 2. Pull the bar down to the level of the breastbone. Then let it release up (while holding bar) and bring it back down for 12 reps. Repeat sequence for 2 sets of 12 reps.

This strengthens the latissimus dorsi muscles of the rib cage and middle back (rhomboids), and secondarily the shoulders and biceps. Strengthening the upper and middle back takes pressure off the lower back.

Slant boards. Avoid them if you have back pain. Keep your chin tucked (to prevent compressing of the cervical verte-brae) while sitting up and lowering down. When you do sit-ups, initiate the movement from underneath the shoulder blades and upper back. Do no pull on your head and neck. If your back hurts, forget the slant board and do your ab exercises on a flat surface. Pay attention to when your back begins to bother you and limit the range of motion to avoid aggravating your back or neck.

Stationary aerobic machines need to be used with the proper body mechanics to prevent back, neck, and knee pain. When using stationary bikes, rowing machines, elliptical riders, cross-country machines, treadmills, and similar equipment, keep your back upright and pelvis tilted. Do not lean forward placing your weight over your hips and onto your arms. This will only strain your back. Stand upright and maintain a neu-tral spine position.

Treadmills continue to be the most popular piece of aer-obic equipment in the home market. Why? You can walk or run, varying the intensity from barely moving to running up a substantial grade. You can gauge your progress and gradu-ally increase to a more challenging level.

The treadmill has many advantages if you suffer from back pain. It keeps your back upright and in the neutral spine position. Plus, the aerobic benefit is excellent in providing circulation of blood to the spine. Rule of thumb: do not use any machines, especially the StairMaster, rowers, or bikes if your back is still hurting. There's too much forward bending, which potentially can strain your back, adding pressure. The NordicTrack, or elliptical trainer, is an excellent nonimpact workout.

Before you work out on ski machines, ellipticals, or Stair-Masters, loosen your ankles. Sit down, and draw several clockwise and counterclockwise circles in the air with your feet, circling the ankles.

Weight lifting accounts for more low back injury than any other sport. This is due to excessive lumbar lordosis (arching).

The key is to maintain trunk control—straight back, knees bent to 80 or 90 degrees max, and pelvis in a tilted position. A belt can be used for more abdominal support and protect the spine.

If you have upper back or neck pain, discontinue using weights until you are completely free of pain. Weights aggravate upper back and neck pain as well as lower back pain. Introduce weights gradually, starting with lower weights and adding two to five pounds incrementally when you are ready. If after the last two reps you struggle to continue, don't add more weight. Wait until the last two reps feel easy. Then you are ready to add weight.

In addition to building and toning muscle, weight lifting reduces stress. When exhaling to push the weight and inhaling to release the movement, your breath is exaggerated and deliberate, which helps reduce stress. If you pace yourself and move from set to set, taking short sixty-second breaks, weight lifting also becomes aerobic, thereby improving the condition of your heart.

On the Field

Baseball is harder on the back than most people realize. It's a real plus to have strong arm muscles and abdominal (core) muscles to prevent the back from straining. Balance and alignment are key to a safe game.

Basketball requires more directional shifts than any other sport. The variety of movements include jumping up to shoot a ball, crouching low to dribble, turning fast for plays, and even taking falls.

Basketball will take its toll on your knees and lower back. However, you can prepare your body for the contortions and falling involved in this sport. Stretch your back, hamstrings, and Achilles muscles before and after the game. Warning: once you tear a hamstring, it could be a year or two before you're back on the court without pain. Never walk onto the court cold, or you'll be crying the blues.

Football players are at greater risk for cervical (neck) injuries than the average person. Head compression injuries are most common. Pads should be used to support the base of the neck. To prevent neck stiffness and permanent injury, I recommend neck strengthening exercises, back stretching and strengthening, and intensive core conditioning.

Golf is an extremely popular sport for both men and women. Many golfers complain of back and neck pain. The reason: weak abdominal (core) muscles, tense back muscles, poor posture, and underconditioned muscles. Plus, the twisting action of a swing places enormous force on the back. Each time you play, you whack the iron with varying velocity over eighty times. The rotation with extension of the spine, which is integral to the golf game, is the culprit.

It is urgent that golfers stay toned in order to decrease their chances of developing back pain. Being in shape can give force to your swing and stamina to your game. It is important to do light or heavy weight lifting to strengthen the arms and shoulders, abdominal exercises for the midsection and core, and squats and lunges for the buttocks (gluteal muscles) and thighs. A powerful swing depends upon these muscle groups working in sync.

Play properly. In order to putt, your back is in a prolonged flexion (forward bending), depending upon the number of balls hit and the length of time spent putting. To prevent back pain, place your hands on your lower back and stretch your back in an extension (back bend). While holding the club in your hands, reach your arms straight up and stretch side to side. Doing this after each swing insures proper alignment and trunk control. Don't forget to maintain awareness of your core muscles, and make an effort to pull them in and up while putting and during all swings.

Also, when bending forward to pick up golf balls, use the proper body mechanics. Never bend over the waist with straight legs. Rather, bend your knees slightly and keep your back upright as you crouch. Or use a suction device on the putter to protect your back, if possible.

The back swing requires extension with rotation. Proper lumbar (low back) alignment must be maintained to prevent lateral bending, which can cause pain when you swing. If you're in pain, cut back on your swing. Stay in the midline area, with your shoulders over the trunk. This will provide more power to your swing. Again, the proper posture is the neutral spine, chest out, chin tucked, pelvic tilt position.

Staying fit, stretching, and maintaining good golf posture will improve performance. Add the aerobic component to your workout and you will feel more energetic, have more endurance, and improve concentration. Prepare your body for the course and enjoy a better game.

Tiger Woods brought an athletic physique to the golf game. The muscles he sculpted through a regimen of heavy lifting were not just appealing to young golfers, they armored him from overusing his back muscles. On April 14, 2019, in an article in *The New York Times*, South African golfer Gary Player spoke about Tiger: "Tiger worked out as if he was a wide receiver or track and field competitor. He was determined to destroy the perception that golfers were not real athletes." After four back surgeries, he was quoted as saying, "I'll never play golf again." Maybe his superstrong, muscular physique saved him from ending his golf career.

Tiger Woods works out at the gym every day, and his physical strength has enabled him to persevere despite his compromised back. His upper body strength, core musculature, and lower body strength have guarded him from overrelying on the back muscles, which twist and torque strenuously during the game.

At age forty-seven, after several back surgeries and with fifteen major titles behind him, Tiger Woods describes himself as a "walking miracle." He is an inspiration to all of us, insisting that his body is top priority. He approaches the course with a finely tuned instrument. It is imperative to condition your body for any athletic endeavor, leisure activity, or simply sitting in a chair.

Tennis is like golf in terms of injury. The most frequent back injuries in tennis occur from playing with cold and/or under-conditioned muscles or bending to pick up the tennis ball incorrectly.

Tennis tune-ups: Use the tennis net to stretch. Hold both hands on the top of the net and walk your body away until your torso is at a right angle to your thighs. This will stretch the shoulders, chest, hamstrings, and calves. Stretch the racket over your head, reaching and twisting the torso right to left. Using full range of motion helps rehearse your tennis muscles.

Jogging and running. Tight joints and poor flexibility are a runner's downfall. Many runners assume that they are stretching their legs through the running motion. This is a myth! Jogging tightens the Achilles tendon, hamstrings, quadriceps, and shins. When you run with tight hamstrings and calves, your hips tighten. Tightness in the hips limits movement. Eventually the tightness will ripple up the spine to either the lower back or neck. Obviously, this affects your stride as well as your pace.

Stretching out the hamstrings (back thighs), Achilles tendons, shins, quadriceps (front thighs), and hips prior to a run is a necessity for running safety.

Joggers and runners who neglect stretching and strengthening the low back have a fifty-fifty chance of back pain. The pounding on the discs can be damaging to the spine. Over time, cartilage and protective cushioning (shock absorbers) between the vertebrae may wear away. If you have back or neck pain, jogging or running are obviously not your best choices.

Skiing, rollerblading, and ice skating all require balance, strength, flexibility, and extreme coordination. The major muscles used are the quadriceps, hamstrings, calves, ankles, and heel cords.

Kamikaze skiers and bladers are risk takers by nature. But the last thing you want to risk is the love of your sport. These sports are all hard on the back. Ligaments in the knees, especially the ACL (anterior cruciate ligament), can twist and tear so quickly you wouldn't know what happened.

You can prepare your body for these sports. Once you take off your ski boots or skates, make sure you lie on your back and stretch the ankles, hamstrings, calves, quads, shins, and back. These sports don't get you in shape. You must approach them with a finely tuned instrument—your body.

The StairMaster, step aerobics, Nautilus equipment, free weights, and stretching each joint will give you a comprehensive workout for skiing, skating, and blading. Consider these pieces of equipment and conditioning as a warmup for your sport.

In the Studio

Dance has many forms and styles. Ballet and jazz dancers often improperly perform the arabesque (back extension and leg lift) and wind up with back pain. Dancers with poor abdominal control and weak psoas muscles (the muscles that connect the pelvis to the thigh) often suffer from back pain as well. Both abdominal and gluteal muscles must be strengthened.

Ballroom dance in general is a wonderful limbering tool. You move every part of your body from your center. Try doing the rhumba without swiveling your hips. Not a chance!

All kinds of dancing—the foxtrot, waltz, merengue, salsa, cha-cha, rumba, and even the sexy tango—enable you to develop form and strength in weakened areas, flexibility in tight joints, and less tension in the shoulders, neck, and back. Dance is therapeutic.

Dancing encourages greater use of the sum of the body parts because the whole body moves naturally with ease. Anyone can transcend their current physical condition this way. When you're dancing, you are using your abdominals, back muscles, calves, thighs, rear end, entire upper body, and your head and neck. You may not be consciously aware of this while you're dancing because it's so enjoyable. That's the best part—the fun part.

If you don't like gyms or formal exercise classes but want to get into shape, try doing the salsa and merengue for an hour. You can make that your cardiovascular workout for the day. Hands down, dancing is my favorite form of fitness exercise. You speak to people when you dance . . . with your body. Besides, think of all the calories you burn off having fun. It's a bargain. If you have arthritis or stiffness in the hips, the merengue is the best Rx in town. It's all hips!

Cross-Train Stretching

Research indicates that it is more effective to address a given muscle group with a variety of exercises. Think about this: do you always train using the same bar or the same lifting routine or go through the same circuit training? I'm suggesting that you mix up your routine for optimum results. You can start by choosing three exercises for each muscle group. Follow the routine for three weeks, then switch to another. In this way you will achieve more strength and power. Variety is the ticket to physical success!

Muscular Strength

Use free weights whenever possible. You may notice how your strength increases. Weights encourage the development of smaller stabilizing muscles and help improve muscular balance and control. Free weights are also versatile because you can work different muscle groups with one set of weights.

If you currently train for strength, consider focusing on your muscular endurance (two sets of twelve to fifteen repetitions, with only short rests between sets), using lighter weights once a week.

For greatest strength gains with heavy weights, emphasize slow movements, especially on the lowering (eccentric) phase. Take at least two seconds to return the weight to its starting position.

Your body performs better when you honor it. If you have a charley horse, do a light workout. Let your muscles rest between sets. Know your limits, and go to a comfortable challenge. Remember, overdoing it is just as bad as underdoing it. Three days a week is just as good as four days a week in terms of strength benefits. Each muscle group needs rest for twenty-four hours to recover.

Work opposing muscle groups on the same day to create balance. For example, if you do chest and back one day, do shoulders, biceps, and triceps the next day. Or work out the upper body one day and lower body the next. If you structure your workouts, you will streamline your time and use it more effectively.

For the greatest results, train at 75 percent to 85 percent of your maximal strength two to three times per week. If your training feels too easy, it's probably resulting in minimal improvements in tone and strength. Don't be afraid to lift a weight five pounds heavier than you are already lifting. Just make sure you have a spotter or a trainer to check for safety and assist you. On heavy days, do six reps at your maximum weight, on medium days do two sets of eight reps at a challenging weight, and on light days do two sets of twelve to fifteen reps using lighter weights.

Treat your body the way you treat your bank account. Like every dollar, every rep counts, and don't give up too soon. Fifty percent of all people who begin an exercise program quit within six months. Fitness fades over time. Taking a two- to four-week break (if not longer) will have a negative effect on the strength gains you've made: the gains you've worked so hard to achieve during the training are lost. Something is better than nothing when it comes to physical activity.

Maintain good posture and alignment while lifting light or heavy weights. Changing positions is fine if the posture remains intact. Start with the pelvic tilt so you have a straight line running through the spine. Think about creating parallel lines even when you're sitting and lifting (head over shoulders, shoulders over hips, hips over knees, keeping the lift in the breastbone.) Most importantly, when you lift weights, activate your abdominals and brace your core. Breathe, breathe, and breathe. Exhale on the exertion. Inhale to release the effort. Use all your energy and your core muscles (not just your arms or legs) to lift the weights. Be conscious of your abs when lifting weights and pull them in toward the spine. Connect your breath to every movement.

Other weight bearing exercise such as walking, hiking, and jogging are effective in building a strong skeletal system. Every time your foot and leg hit the ground, you send a vibration up the leg. This strengthens the bones and may prevent osteopenia and osteoporosis.

Weight lifting reduces stress and improves your sense of personal power and confidence, positive body esteem, and mood. As you progress, you receive a feeling of reaching your goals both in and out of the gym. Two strength training workouts per week is ideal.

Cross–Train Stretching

Cross-train stretching is sports-specific training used as a conditioning tool for multimuscular activities. Stretching takes the straitjacket off your body. The goal is to elongate the spine, expand through the chest, and extend through every joint in your body as you stretch. In order to untense your back, neck and shoulder muscles, it's optimal to stretch most days of the week. If you are pressed for time, even five or ten minutes will be of great benefit.

Ideally, you should stretch after all of your workouts and on your days off. The movement of stretching is outward. Stretch, hold the stretch, relax, breathe, and lengthen . . . and risk stretching a little further. Gently prod your body to the next level of stretch that your body can receive. Stop after each stretch and notice the effects. Remember, over-stretching is just as dangerous as understretching. Go easy, or you might tear a tight muscle. This is not a competition. Don't compare yourself to people younger than yourself, older than yourself, or even yourself when you were younger. Simply start from where your body is today, accept it with all its flaws, and work toward greater flexibility! Stretch at your own pace.

I've heard many people complain that they don't want to stretch because it'll diminish their strength gains. This is a myth. The more flexible you are, the greater range of motion you have to lift weights.

Stretching tunes you into your sixth, kinesthetic sense: the subtle sensation of your body in stillness or motion. My bodyformula fitness philosophy is: *Be as flexible as you are strong!*

Breathe properly. Breathe from your belly, not your chest. Place your hands on your belly; as you breathe in deeply through your nose, feel the belly inflate like a balloon. As you exhale, feel the belly deflate as if letting air out of a balloon. As you hold the stretch, you inhale through the nostrils, with lips sealed if you can. This form of breathing (yoga breathing) allows your lungs to take in seven times more oxygen. As you exhale, release the air slowly through your nostrils.

Reach and stretch. Set aside ten minutes a day for energy stretching. Start your day with stretching to infuse your body with oxygen and energy. End your day with stretching to release pent-up tension, distorted postures, and stress. When you stretch a little bit each day, you diminish the damaging effects of accumulated mental and physical fatigue. You create a feeling of vitality and balance. It's better than a cup of coffee!

Stretch at work. Get up and take a stretch break every forty-five minutes to an hour to reduce back and neck pain, drooping keyboard posture, and carpal tunnel syndrome. Stretch your fingers and hands daily.

Stretch after sports. A little prevention goes a long way. Use stretching for the tune-ups before basketball, tennis, golf, dancing, and similar activities. Before or after each swing of your club or bat, stretch your back, shoulders, and entire trunk. A hip flexor stretch will liberate the tightness from walking, twisting, and repetitive forward bending (see hip flexor stretch at end of chapter). Stretch after all physical activities. Taut muscles work much less efficiently and will stop your growth toward peak performance.

When muscles remain tight, you can pull a muscle, tendon, or a ligament. Why? The explanation is simple. Ligaments connect muscle to muscle and surrounding joints. If the ligaments are not flexible, you'll strain the muscle. Something has to give. Like a tight rubber band, the ligament can snap when you least expect it. It'll set you back weeks, if not months. Stretching can help prevent calcium deposits, tendinitis, and arthritis. When you stop moving and stretching, you lose your youthful appearance. Regardless of age, stretching helps maintain an easygoing, agile stride.

With sports or any physical activity, when the spine is overarched or overstretched, it's easy to throw your back out. Luckily, simply tucking the pelvis under limits the strain placed on the back. Once finished with your sport, a simple solution to relax your back is to use pillows under your knees if you are lying on your back, or between the knees if you are lying on the side.

Tools for Stretching

Use a rope. You can buy a rope at any hardware store or a yoga strap at a sporting goods store. Now lie on your back and place the rope around the ball of your foot. Flex and point the foot to stretch the heel cord (Achilles tendon). Then straighten the knee so the leg is long and bring the rope (with your leg) toward your face to stretch the hamstring. Repeat on the other leg.

Stretching Know–How

Stay still. Hold the stretch and breathe into it. Ballistic stretching (where you pulse or bounce over a muscle) makes the muscles recoil. Don't do it.

Active isolation (AI stretching). Stretch one muscle at a time. The opposing muscle will automatically contract. Hold the position for two to three seconds, then release and restretch. What happens is, you increase your stretch little by little. It's a good idea to look for a trainer who is qualified in AI stretching.

Stretching can expand you both physically and mentally. Don't swear by any one method. Keep exploring all the techniques until you find one that feels right. Stretch your body and mind. Together they won't sag with age!

Water Exercise

Whether you play a sport such as golf, tennis, soccer, baseball, or basketball, take exercise classes, lift weights, jog, dance, spin, or are sedentary (deconditioned) or injured through sports or an accident, water exercise is key!

Hard-core exercise is great . . . to a point. It's imperative to balance your sport activities. The physiological properties of an aquatic environment are especially good for the back, neck, and all the joints. The body is 90 percent buoyant in water, leaving 10 percent body weight. This allows for increased mobility while mitigating pain.

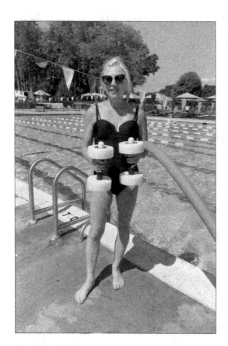 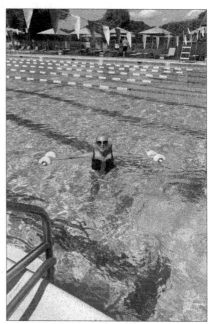

Water Workout

Step 1. Have a water noodle and buoys with you before you enter a shallow pool. In a deep-water pool, a buoyancy belt provides total body support.

Step 2. Before entering deep water, place a noodle in between legs, like riding a horse. Get into the water, then take the water buoys in each hand. Your body is now buoyant. Submerge the buoys down to the hips. Begin walking laps up and down the pool. The noodle or buoyancy belt will allow your feet to lift off the pool floor, providing total buoyancy. Walk in the water as if you are walking on land for at least 20 minutes. Extend arms and legs in opposition as you walk. This relaxes all the joints and provides upper body resistance with the buoys. It is a challenging cardiovascular workout as well as conditioning the upper and lower body.

Walking in the water is relatively easy. The water will support your body weight, enabling you to feel light and flexible. You can increase the resistance by using water buoys (weights). The water weights vary between ten and forty pounds, depending upon how hard you are working. Water noodles are helpful as well if you don't have a buoyancy belt. While walking and pushing or pulling a noodle, you will feel a light resistance in your arms and upper back without straining your lower back or neck. You can also wear a buoyancy belt around your midsection and walk in deep water. This takes the pressure off the knees, feet, and ankles without pounding the floor of the pool. Gravity is no longer an issue and will relax the back profoundly.

Walking in the water is an easy way to begin to move. Submerging the head underwater (for a few seconds) is a way to clear the cobwebs. This has a therapeutic effect for headaches and neck pain.

Aqua exercise is an excellent holistic remedy for the wrists, hands, and fingers as well. Whether you have carpal tunnel syndrome or repetitive strain injury or suffer from tingling and numbness in the forearms, wrists, or hands, the buoyancy of the water allows for increased circulation and blood flow. While walking in the water, glide the hands while pronating and supinating (turning the wrists and hands forward and backward) with the fingers separated. This has a soothing effect on the wrists, hands, fingers, forearms, and shoulders. Water therapy is also known to improve the mood.

Ideally, water exercise should be done in a warm-water, indoor pool, five to seven times per week to alleviate joint aches and pain. Sessions should last for thirty to sixty minutes. If it is difficult to walk on land because of a back or neck injury, try it in water. You will be amazed how easily you move and without pain.

Quick Cures Following
Exercise-Induced Injuries

In emergency episodes of acute pain, follow these instructions. *If any of the steps cause you pain, stop immediately!*

Stop! Lie on the floor with your rear close to the legs of a chair and place calves on the seat of the chair, (see photo, chapter 1).

Rest! Don't exercise for one day. The next day, lie flat on your back and do a few small pelvic tilts every two hours (see photo, chapter 1). Roll onto your belly and do a few slow back push-ups every few hours, but only if this position does not cause pain. If it does, discontinue this movement and do only pelvic tilts.

Relax! Breathe mindfully. Take a few deep breaths and exhale slowly. Repeat the following words silently: relax . . . be still . . . be calm.

Aspirin, ice, and heating pads. Consult with your doctor first. Aspirin, ibuprofen, or Aleve take down the swelling and relieve the pain. Anti-inflammatories can be extremely useful during the acute phase. Then apply ice packs for twenty minutes every hour until the pain subsides. Follow with alternating cold and heat (nonelectric heating pads are best).

Alternative methods. Homeopathy, acupuncture, herbs, and massage all provide excellent healing properties. Back yourself up with resources.

After the pain. Start a program of exercise to build up your back and abdominal (core) muscles and ample stretching to increase flexibility. Don't get caught in trouble again!

Broom Stick Stretches

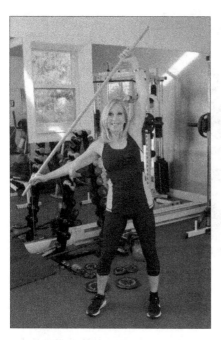 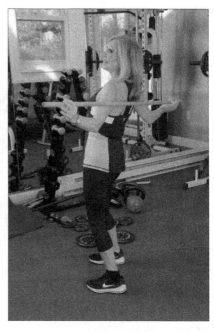

Step 1. Hold a broomstick at the ends. Lift it above the head while stretching both arms straight. Reach the upper body to the right, then to the left. 12 reps. This improves upper body flexibility and improves posture.

Step 2. Reach the broomstick above head and lower it behind the upper back. If you have restricted range of motion, attempt the end position to increase flexibility. Eventually you can work the broomstick behind upper back. This improves posture as the shoulders open and the chest (pectoral) muscles stretch. Think of stretching a tight rubber band.

Upper Body Strength Training

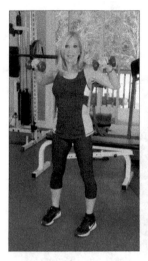 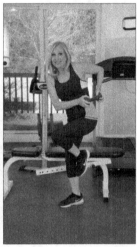 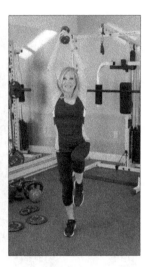

Step 1. Stand with feet hip distance apart in good standing posture. Hold one weight in each hand. Bring weights to the shoulders. Lift both weights straight up to the ceiling until elbows straighten.

Step 2. Return the weights to shoulders. Repeat shoulder presses for 12 reps. Use weights that feel challenging but not impossible. It should feel challenging but not impossible.

Step 1. Hold one weight with both hands.

Step 2. Bend one knee and lift it up toward chest while twisting the weight behind the waistline. Return foot to floor after each rep. Repeat this for 24 reps on each side. This tones the waistline and increases mobility in the spine.

Step 1. Stand with feet hip distance apart, and hold weight at the center with both hands.

Step 2. Lift the weight above your head, then bend elbows to lower weight behind your head.

Step 3. Straighten both arms so weight is straight above the head. Alternating lifting one thigh high up toward chest at a time.

Repeat sequence for 16 reps.

Core Strength

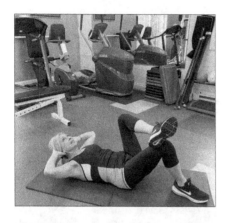

Step 1. Lie flat on the floor with lower back pressed into a mat. Place hands behind the head and lift the head and shoulders off the floor.

Step 2. Lift one leg up and place the foot on the opposite knee.

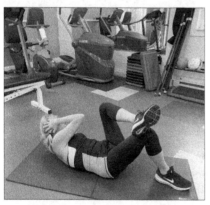

Step 3. Lift opposite shoulder and elbow to reach across the body toward the opposite knee.

Step 4. Return arm and shoulder to start position. Repeat this for 12 reps. Then switch sides and repeat the sequence.

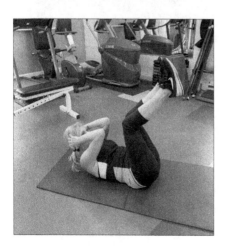

Start position: lie flat on the floor with feet touching the mat, head on floor, with hands behind the head.

Step 1. Raise bent knees up and over the chest, and lift lower legs to ceiling. Simultaneously lift shoulders and bent arms off the floor and up toward the knees. Exhale as you lift. Then lower feet to floor; lower shoulders and elbows to floor as well. Inhale through the nose as you lower down. This works core muscles. Repeat for 12 reps.

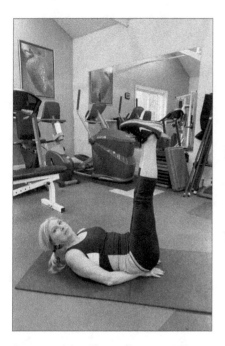 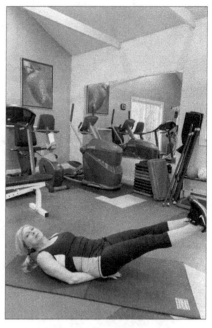

Start position: lie on floor and lift hips up to place both hands (palms down) under lower back. This protects the back from arching, prevents back pain, and helps locate the core muscles.

Step 1. Lower legs to hover 6 inches off floor.

Step 2. Then raise the legs back up toward ceiling. Repeat 8–16 reps, depending upon core strength. If your back hurts, do not lower the legs more than a few inches toward the floor.

Hip Flexor Stretch

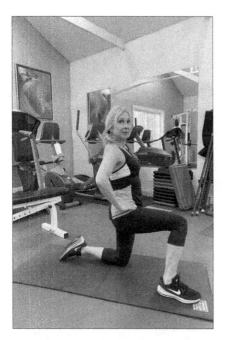 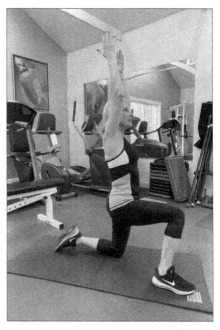

Knee pain sufferers should avoid this sequence.

Step 1. Drop down to one knee on a cushioned mat. Step forward with front leg. Use good posture and lift the chest up; roll shoulders back and down.

Step 2. Place hands on hips and press pelvis forward. This stretches the hip flexor of the back thigh, the iliopsoas muscle. Repeat the same exercise on the other side. Hold each position 8–12 seconds for maximum lengthening.

Same starting position as step 1 (left). Maintain good posture with chin in, breastbone lifted, and pelvis thrusting forward. Lift both arms straight up and overhead. Hold position 8–12 seconds.

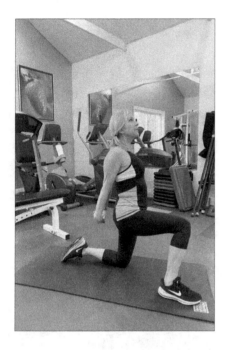

Same starting position as on page 149.

Step 1. Clasp both arms behind the back.

Step 2. Lift arms up and away from back with straight elbows. This stretches the hip flexor and posture muscles of the chest and rotator cuffs. Hold the position 8–12 seconds.

Posture Perfected

Start position: Stand with feet hip distance apart and in good posture. Chin in, breastbone and back of the head lifted.

Step 1. Place both hands behind the head and open the elbows, pulling the arms back while squeezing the shoulder blades (scapulae) together in midback area.

This improves three postural misalignments: kyphosis (rounded shoulders), lordosis (back arching), and scoliosis (lateral curvature of the spine.)

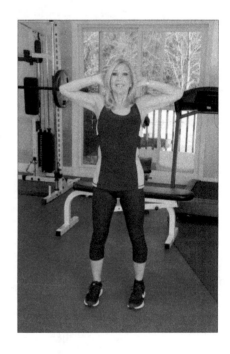

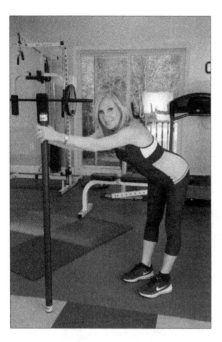 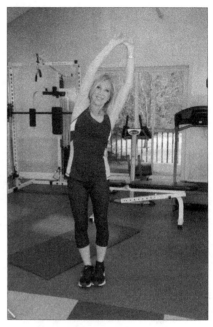

Body Bar Stretch

Start position: stand tall and hold a body bar toward the top end with both hands.

Step 1. Walk your feet away from the bar and keep the arms outstretched to form a perpendicular angle with the upper torso and legs.

Step 2. Press chest forward and downward toward floor. This stretches the hamstrings, gluteal muscles of the buttocks, lower back, and shoulders.

Step 3. Bring the body bar in toward chest, and arch the back as the chest lifts up toward ceiling. Repeat this sequence 3 times.

Spine Stretch

The Spine Stretch can be done at home, the gym, or work to reverse the seated position. It may reduce back pain if done regularly.

Start position: stand with feet and ankles close together.

Step 1. Interlace the thumbs, and stretch both arms up to the ceiling.

Step 2. Press hips to one side and stretch arms to the opposite side. Hold the position 8 seconds. Repeat on the other side. Come back to start position.

This elongates the spine and stretches from the hip to the end of the fingertips on each side.

Chapter 8
How to Stay Motivated

The only thing you can control is how hard you
are willing to work for your physical goals.
—CARL LEWIS, WORLD-CLASS ATHLETE
AND OLYMPIC GOLD MEDALIST

Your lifestyle can affect your lifespan. Staying active and eating a healthy diet is crucial to living longer and healthier. Nutritious meals, ample exercise, and stress reduction constitute a healthy lifestyle.

Most people complain that they need to lose five pounds or more. Diets don't always work, as you will eventually go off the diet. Try to avoid any diet that eliminates an entire food group; otherwise, eventually cravings and the feeling of deprivation take over and weaken resolve to stay on the diet. Rigid, complicated diets don't work on a long-term basis. Anyone can lose weight for a short period of time on a diet, often eliminating an entire food group, but this often leads to recidivism: weight regained, plus a few extra pounds.

The best way to lose weight is by maintaining a healthy diet and exercising five to seven times per week for forty-five minutes to one hour each day. Don't forget to add a yoga class at least once a week to reinforce deep breathing, stretching, and relaxation techniques. The regular practice of yoga will help control your level of stress.

The following is a basic, flexible eating plan. Hopefully, it is one that you can live with comfortably. I hesitate to state food rules, as rules are easily broken. Rather, these are broad guidelines you can adhere to and still enjoy your lifestyle.

Breakfast is the most important meal. According to diabetes expert Amy Campbell, "when you wake up, blood sugar levels are low. Eating breakfast helps to stabilize blood sugar levels." "Breaking the fast" gets your metabolism going. If you skip breakfast, you slow down your metabolism, which may lead to weight gain. Distributing calories evenly throughout the day regulates the metabolism. Eating breakfast revs up your metabolism first thing in the morning. Food stimulates your body.

Make sure you eat something in the morning, even if you don't have an appetite for breakfast. A banana, a breakfast bar, or protein shake will do the trick occasionally. Breakfast is brain food and wakes up the brain and the body to function optimally. Remember, if it's good for the body, it's good for the brain.

Sample breakfasts: two to three eggs, any style; omelettes are great, as you can add vegetables, such as scallions, spinach, mushrooms, and peppers. Replace whole milk with almond milk or cashew milk. Add Greek yogurt or nondairy yogurt with berries to your breakfast, as these are excellent sources of protein and fruit. High-fiber dry cereal or oat-meal, two to three times per week, are important sources of fiber. Smoothies are a great breakfast drink. A simple rec-ipe is frozen strawberries, frozen bananas, almond milk, and coconut milk. Flax seeds, hemp, and a dollop of Greek yogurt are optional. You can add small amounts of honey, agave, or maple syrup. Variety, rather than eating the same thing every day, is the key to eating healthy meals.

Sample lunch: Salad is a great option. Make sure you add as many vegetables as possible: lettuce; tomatoes; cucumbers; scallions; mushrooms; green, red, yellow, or orange peppers; hot peppers; broccoli; avocado; beets. Walnuts, almonds, sunflower seeds, pumpkin seeds, and Brazil nuts are the healthiest nuts. You can toss them in salad or eat them as a snack. Adding a protein such as grilled chicken, fish, tofu, eggs, cottage cheese, or lean meat will provide energy. Pro-tein gives you energy, while carbohydrates induce fatigue. One slice of bread is ample (if it is whole-grain bread, not white bread). Gluten-free bread and products are widely sold if you are restricted to a gluten-free diet.

Salad dressing: mix olive oil, balsamic vinegar, Dijon mustard, lemon, and a pinch of salt and pepper for flavor. Use store-bought or restaurant dressing sparingly, and read the labels when available.

Grill your chicken and fish. Salmon is a great choice. Avoid all fried foods. Say no to fried chicken and French fries. Refined carbohydrates; white bread, white rice and white sugar spike your blood sugar quickly and are stored in the fat cells. Try to avoid all white carbohydrates as much as possible.

Whole grains—brown rice, sweet potatoes, quinoa, buckwheat (kasha), and steel-cut oatmeal—are healthy carbohydrates. They are slow-burning grains and won't raise your blood sugar too high. They contain fiber, which is good for digestion.

Eat plenty of fruit: apples, pears, banana, mango, pineapple, and berries (strawberries, blueberries, blackberries, and raspberries) are sweet and delicious and full of antioxidants. Fill half your plate with red, yellow, and green vegetables every day. The more colorful your plate, the healthier it is. Eat or drink vegetables in abundance. Vegetable juices count!

Cake, candy, and ice cream should be avoided unless eaten in moderation. A small amount, around 150–200 calories, is a reasonable dessert. This may sound impossible, but try sharing a dessert instead of eating the whole thing alone. Look for healthy dessert recipes. One small piece of dark chocolate for dessert, applesauce, or baked apples are healthy choices. Dried fruit: apricots, figs, dates, raisins, and cranberries are also good choices in small amounts. Remember to read labels and note the portion size for the allotted calories. You may be shocked at the calorie count for a small amount. For instance, three dried apricots are fifty calories. Calories are sneaky and quickly add up.

Chips are dangerous, as you can easily lose count and consume an entire bag before the blink of an eye. I suggest you eat fifteen chips max, then quit. Be supervigilant and conscious about your snack and dessert calories. These empty calories add up quickly. Anyone allergic to wheat or gluten must follow the advice of their physician.

You can maintain a good diet even at restaurants. However, there are a few obstacles. A basket of bread placed in front of you while you are waiting for your meal is tantalizing and can kill the appetite. Consuming empty calories to the tune of 200–500 extra calories or more quickly adds up to a pound or two weight gain in one week. Before you turn around, a few pounds creep on, especially if you are over forty years old and not that active. Push the bread basket away and enjoy your meal. Make healthier eating choices, challenge yourself physically, and be more active every day.

Whether you choose to lose weight to improve your back pain or fit better in your clothes, a substantial weight loss will improve your overall health and help create a positive attitude and improved body esteem. Losing weight will take the axial load off the spine and reduce back and neck pain and hip, knee, and ankle pain. You may want to work with a registered dietitian to create an individualized eating plan you can adhere to. Sometimes having someone to check in with keeps you accountable for your healthy dietary efforts.

Once you begin to exercise regularly, you will have more vigor and energy. Energy creates more energy, and this becomes contagious. Your metabolism will improve, and you are more apt to eat healthier meals. Your mood will improve, and you will feel entirely different. Movement is the key to healthy living, and it's never too late to improve your fitness level and your diet. Make small, incremental changes, and notice how much better you feel. Choose an apple over a brownie or take the stairs instead of the elevator; walk around the block after dinner instead of sinking into the couch. The small decisions we make every day create the greatest impact over time.

In a lecture entitled "Harness the Power of Exercise on Your Brain," neuroscientist Wendy A. Suzuki, PhD, a professor at New York University, states that physical activity transforms your brain. Aerobic exercise such as walking, for example, improves your mood and ability to focus. Dr. Suzuki reports that exercise also reduces depression, hostility, and anxiety and can be more effective than antidepressants.

The hippocampus is the section of the brain that stores long-term memory and is most affected by exercise. With exercise, new brain cells, which are critical for long-term memory, grow within the hippocampus. Getting fit improves brain function.

My bodyformula method is to establish an exercise routine almost every day and manage all aspects of health and well-being. It involves a connection between the mind and the body. It requires being disciplined about scheduling your workouts and keeping the appointments. Any aerobic activity that gets your pulse rate up to between 60 to 85 percent of your maximum heart rate and keeps it there for thirty minutes to one hour will have significant cardiac benefit and reduce stress. However, if you only have ten, twenty, or thirty minutes, it is better than nothing. Walking thirty to sixty minutes every day pays off twice: you will walk off a couple of pounds per month at the very least and reduce stress. Walking is the single best exercise for a bad back, as you are upright, which maintains the neutral spine position. You can monitor your pain level as you walk on land or in the water. If you are in pain, stop the activity rather than pushing past the pain. That will backfire.

Break a sweat three to six times per week to assure that your workouts are optimally beneficial. This raises the metabolism, making your muscles metabolically more active even at rest.

As stated earlier, water exercise is the best workout for anyone with joint pain or arthritis or recovering from an injury. It also balances out hard-core exercise and makes the chore of working out more pleasant by not straining the joints. Using water equipment such as a noodle, water buoys (weights), and a buoyancy belt will provide resistance for a challenging workout. Search for a gym or YMCA with an indoor pool for year-round exercise.

If you want to live without back pain as you age, strength training is key! Then you won't over rely on wiry back muscles. The aging body needs strength training, as we lose muscle and bone density every year without it. Include two to four strength training workouts per week to strengthen your muscles and bones and prevent osteoporosis. Use light weights (between one and ten pounds) to strengthen your upper body. As you progress, gradually add weight. Studies have found that even people in their nineties benefit from strength training two to three times per week.

There is no magic bullet. Diet, exercise, and stress reduction are inextricably intertwined. It's so important to pay attention to what you eat, as you can't outtrain a poor diet. All the exercise in the world cannot make up for a nutrient-poor, high-calorie diet.

At bodyformula gym with clients.

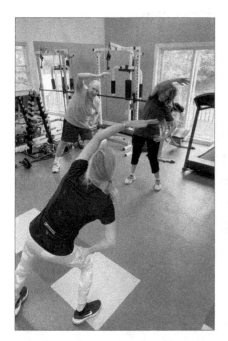
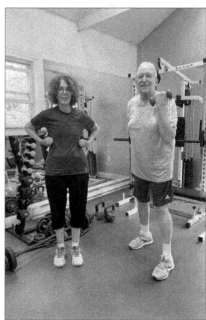
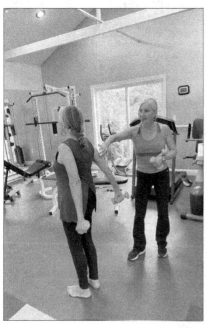
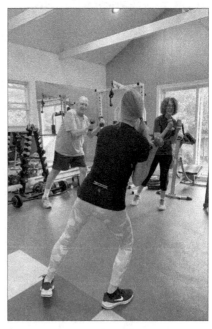

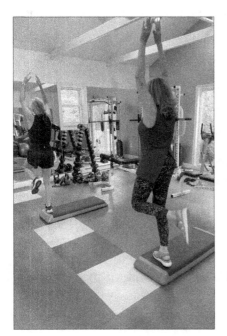
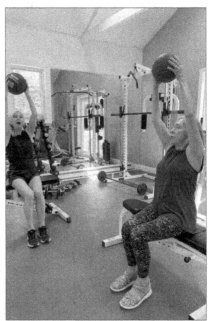

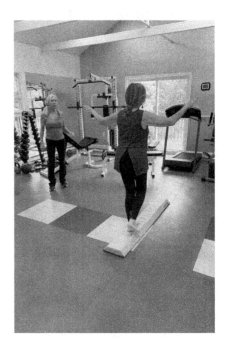

Balance Routine

Stand with good posture, chin in, breastbone lifted, arms at sides or on hips. Walk with one foot in front of the other. Keep the head up and eyes looking straight in front, not down. This improves balance and should be practiced daily.

To improve eating habits, keep it simple—isolate one unhealthy habit at a time and make changes incrementally. For instance, instead of eating dessert every night, cut back to once or twice a week or switch from cake and ice cream to fruit, nuts and/or a small piece of dark chocolate.

Know your trigger foods, and uncover which foods lead to uncontrollable cravings. If you favor salty foods or sweets, limit your intake. Read food labels! Calories count, but total carbohydrate count is key.

Meal preparation every week will sharpen your resolve to improve your diet. Shop for healthy, easy to grab food for your fridge. When you open the door, you can grab healthy prepared foods galore. Make a pot of quinoa, cut up mushrooms, cucumber slices, red and yellow peppers, sprinkle in dried cranberries and pine nuts if you like them. Healthy food can be delicious!

Be supervigilant in restaurants. Follow the no-bread rule unless you can discipline yourself to eat the crust of one piece of bread. One glass of wine for women, two glasses for men. Share one dessert, three to four bites max. Don't let your hard-earned lost pounds creep up!

Exercise is medicine and is essential for good health, well-being, and weight loss. It should be done on a long-term basis. You simply can't coast on workouts you've had previous weeks, months, or years. Rather than thinking about what you used to do when you were younger, focus on what you can do today. Try not to procrastinate and get moving right away. You are never too old to get into shape!

Tip Sheet: Strategies for a Healthy Lifestyle

1. Control your portions and keep track of calories as they add up quickly. Think moderation!
2. Be mindful when you eat. Avoid overeating when bored, tired, or stressed.
3. Exercise 150 minutes per week. Ample exercise burns calories, reduces stress, and helps controls back pain.
4. Check the scale no more than once a week or once a month. Don't become a slave to the scale.
5. Keep a food log. Monitoring your food intake ensures success.
6. Get started right away with exercise and healthy diet and avoid procrastination.
7. Find a buddy to exercise with to ensure adherence. Walk, run, and lift weights.
8. Don't eat past 8 p.m. on weeknights and around 9 p.m. on weekends, when you normally go to bed later. Leave one and a half to two hours before sleep to digest.
9. Break a sweat three times per week minimum. Aerobic exercise and strength training burns fat and raise the metabolism.
10. Remain calm and carry on. Optimism is the best attitude.

I have dedicated my life to helping people get strong backs, clear minds, and healthy lifestyles. Please enjoy a trip down my memory lane of fitness coaching below. Let it inspire and motivate you to create your own healthy life memories, no matter your age! If you are inspired toward a healthy lifestyle, congratulations: you're back on track.

Follow: bodyformulafitness on Instagram for exercise on the go.

Visit www.bodyformula.com to view my fitness blog and video clips.

Acknowledgments

would like to acknowledge my husband, Alex, retired general surgeon and hand surgeon of fifty years. He encouraged me to write this book while I was pregnant with our son, David. He provided his medical expertise for those chapters which involved the anatomy and function of the back and wrists.

To my children, Vanessa and David, who brighten my life. I want to thank my daughter Vanessa for her unwavering support and technical expertise . . . and for our meaningful conversations at all hours of the day and night. I want to thank my son David for his unending support and positive attitude in our family. David has been a guiding light for our family. I am thrilled to have this book completed for Vanessa and David to cherish.

I want to thank Diane Rosano for her creative marketing expertise with my book and for providing many of its featured photos, and for producing and managing my social media and website content. She offered vital input and guidance at a crucial time in the development and completion of the book for which I am very grateful. I want to also thank Diane's husband, Joel Rosano, for his technical expertise regarding my manuscript and for providing some exceptional photographs.

I'd like to thank Mike Share of Color Magic Inc., for building my website and logo design and providing ongoing support and input during many planning meetings over the years.

I thank Elaine Heimberger for her editing expertise and for the title of the book. Elaine edited the book in its final phase. Her patience, and many hours of editing and helping me focus my thoughts, were invaluable.

I'd like to thank Seth Gershel, publishing consultant, for his many hours of publishing expertise and marketing guidance. Seth was vice president of audiobooks at Simon & Schuster for eighteen years. His belief in my success keeps me going—enabling me to see the light at the end of the tunnel. Seth has spent many hours advising me with my four DVDs and my book over the years, for which I am grateful.

I thank Bill Waltzer, photographer, www.waltzer.com, for his photographs. In addition to his photography business, Bill was an adjunct professor at CW Post LIU, teaching photojournalism.

I thank photojournalist Ken Kerbs for the photographs of his daily back exercise routine, and Ingrid Belqaid for her photography. I also thank Paulo Pinheiro, personal trainer, owner of Personal Training Studio, Exercise Excellence in Tucson, Arizona, for the photos of his well-defined back muscles.

I send gratitude to Aubrey Swartz, MD, orthopedic surgeon and former director of the American Back Society. He gave me the platform to perform my exercise classes to conference members for seven years while attending ABS conventions. I was also fortunate to attend the conferences and receive 200 hours of continuing medical education on the spine and back care. I had the honor of presenting my back exercise program to American Back Society conference members (including physicians, chiropractors, physical therapists and other health care professionals) in conjunction with physical therapist Carol McFarland, PT, as part of the convention curriculum.

Bibliography

Benson, Herbert, MD. *The Relaxation Response*. Rev. ed. New York: Morrow, 2000.

Feldenkrais, Moshe. *The Master Moves*. Cupertino, CA.: Meta Publications, 1984.

Marcus, Norman, MD. *End Back Pain Forever*. New York: Atria, 2012.

Nitti, Joseph T., MD, and Kimberlie Nitti. *The Interval Training Workout*. Nashville, TN.: Hunter House, 2001.

Sarno, John, MD. *The Mind Body Prescription: Healing the Body, Healing the Mind*. New York: Warner, 1998.

———. *Mind over Back Pain*. New York: Morrow, 1982.

Schubert, Keith W., MD. *Stress/Unstress: How You Can Control Stress at Home and on the Job*. Minneapolis: Augsburg, 1981.

Selye, Hans. *Stress in Health and Disease*. Boston: Butterworth/Heinemann, 2013.

Stough, Carl, and Reece Stough. *Dr. Breath: The Story of Breathing Coordination*. New York: Morrow, 1970.

About the Author

Roberta Bergman is founder of Roberta's Bodyformula™, a wellness program for individuals committed to improving their overall health through fitness, proper nutrition and back pain prevention.

As an ACE certified Fitness Instructor and WaterArt International certified Aqua Instructor,

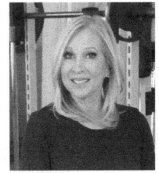

Photo by Bill Waltzer

Roberta also holds an M.S. in Movement Therapy. With her extensive training and work experience, Roberta is often asked to lecture on ways to relieve back pain which includes medically safe exercise, posture perfected movement and healthy lifestyle choice.

Please visit www.bodyformula.com and @bodyformula fitness on Instagram, to learn more about Roberta.

Printed in the USA
CPSIA information can be obtained
at www.ICGtesting.com
JSHW012326281223
54480JS00003B/22